THE THINKING
MOMS' REVOLUTION

"Don't judge each day by the harvest you reap
but by the seeds you plant."
—ROBERT LOUIS STEVENSON

THE THINKING
MOMS' REVOLUTION

AUTISM BEYOND THE SPECTRUM: INSPIRING TRUE STORIES FROM PARENTS FIGHTING TO RESCUE THEIR CHILDREN

COLLECTED BY
HELEN CONROY AND **LISA JOYCE GOES**

Skyhorse Publishing

Skyhorse Publishing books may be purchased in bulk at special discounts for sales promotion, corporate gifts, fund-raising, or educational purposes. Special editions can also be created to specifications. For details, contact the Special Sales Department, Skyhorse Publishing, 307 West 36th Street, 11th Floor, New York, NY 10018 or info@skyhorsepublishing.com.

Skyhorse® and Skyhorse Publishing® are registered trademarks of Skyhorse Publishing, Inc.®, a Delaware corporation.

Visit our website at www.skyhorsepublishing.com.

10 9 8 7 6 5 4 3

Library of Congress Cataloging-in-Publication Data is available on file.
ISBN: 978-1-62087-884-2

Printed in the United States of America

To the revolutionaries who carved the path before us; to all the Thinking Moms and Dads who keep us moving forward each day; and to our children, whom we will carry to the finish line of health, healing, and recovery. We love you.

CONTENTS

FOREWORD

Autism. Let me say it again: Autism. How does that word make you feel? What emotions does it bring out? Fear? Sympathy? Empathy? Autism. But it's not just a word. If only it could simply be a word in a medical dictionary that describes a neurodevelopmental disorder that affects 1 in 10,000 children. That's what autism used to be. It didn't affect your family. It didn't affect your neighbor's child. Autism wasn't on your street, and it probably wasn't even in your zip code. Autism was in a movie, and that was about it.

So what the freaking hell happened?

Autism is now in your family. It's on your block. It's a child in every kindergarten class. There are entire classrooms devoted to autism in every public school. Autism is no longer just a word; it's life for over a million people in the United States. And it isn't pretty. There's nothing glamorous about raising a child with autism. It's brutal. It tears families apart, after it bankrupts them. Autism. One percent of children have it. Two percent of boys have it. Autism can no longer be ignored.

Ignored? Who the hell would ignore such a problem? The American medical community, that's who. When autism exploded in the 1990s, parents cried out for help. These children needed treatment, but insurance didn't cover it. These parents wanted answers, and doctors said "Answers to what? There's no rise in autism, and there's nothing we can really do for it anyway, so what do you want *us* to do about it?" Parents were literally left to fend for themselves to find answers and treatment options—alone. If there is one word that accurately describes families who were caught up in the first wave of the autism epidemic, it is *alone*. Alone with no answers, no friends, no cures, and no resources.

Well, nothing brings about change like a group of dedicated parents who are fighting for their own children. The Thinking

Moms' Revolution is one such group, and boy, are they on fire! And they have a story to tell. Twenty-three stories, in fact. And they are not just about autism. You will read about ADHD, dyspraxia, sensory processing disorder, and other learning and developmental challenges. You, and I, and every person on the planet has a responsibility to hear their stories. Not for *their* benefit, but for yours. For mine. We owe it to ourselves to experience, page by agonizing page, what a family goes through when they see their happy, healthy, talkative little toddler lose it all and decline into autism. The denial. The anger. The guilt.

Why? Why should *you* care what *they* went through? Of course, if you just found out that your own child has autism, you probably care a great deal, and you are eager to soak up every page. But what about the rest of us? What about the 87 out of 88 of us who *don't* have a child with autism? Why should you care? Because this book will make you examine your own understanding of autism. It will challenge what you believe causes, or doesn't cause, autism. It will illuminate the myriad treatment options that are available. But most importantly, it will make *you* a better person. Next time you are in the grocery store and see a six-year-old nonverbal child having a complete meltdown, instead of frowning and thinking what a bad job that parent is doing, you can go up to them and say, "I get it. I don't have a child with autism, so I don't totally get it. But I'm trying. Can I give you a helping hand?" When your best friend's toddler begins flapping, spinning, and obsessing about trains, you can stick by them, love them, and help guide them through the coming years because you've learned empathy. When your own child tells you that his friend in third grade seems a little strange and talks funny, you can teach your child how to love unconditionally as you befriend and embrace that family.

The Thinking Moms' Revolution isn't looking for sympathy, and neither is any other family with autism. If you want to sympathize and shed a tear for them, do so, then get over it. Once you are done, step up and love them. Embrace them. Engage them. Not for their benefit, but for yours. And you will have plenty of opportunity to empathize, as autism continues to rise at an alarming rate.

The latest numbers (1 in 88) aren't actually the latest numbers at all. This statistic is 13 years old. It refers to children who were born in the year 2000. Back in the '80s it was 1 in 10,000. Then wham! Kids born in 1994 were found to have a rate of autism of 1 in 150. Nobody panicked (except about 1 in 150 of us). Kids born in 1998 were found to have a rate of 1 in 110. You do the math. What do you think the rate is for kids born in 2004? 2008? 2013? The Centers for Disease Control only determines the rate for a certain year once that group is eight years old. Then it takes a couple years to gather the data and publish it. So, we won't actually have numbers for 2013 until somewhere around the year 2023.

As a full-time practicing pediatrician, I can vouch without a shred of doubt that the rate continues to rise. I see more and more seemingly healthy infants develop autism signs during the second year of life. It concerns me that the rate is now much higher than 1 in 88. And we still don't know why. You will read various opinions from the Thinking Moms here, but based on available research, we just don't yet know why. What angers me is that the medical community should have started examining this question twenty years ago. Instead, (almost) all put their heads in the sand and decided there was no increase, there was no epidemic, so there is no reason to examine why. Now that everyone agrees there is a definite increase, research into what's causing autism has begun. I know we'll find the answer some day, but it's an answer that will come twenty years later than it should have.

In the meantime, what can we do? We can detect it early, so that early treatment can increase the chance of recovery. We can embrace complementary and alternative treatments that work. We can take some preventive steps with our health before and during pregnancy, and during the first years of a baby's life. We can do the best we can to treat each and every child with autism to the best of our abilities. And we can love these children, and their mommies and daddies. We can understand what these children go through during their years of therapy, what their parents go through emotionally and financially, and how these families fight for their children to get them to where they are today.

The Thinking Moms' Revolution's *Autism Beyond the Spectrum* is a look into the hearts and minds of these families. After reading their stories, you will want to hunt each one of them down, give them a big hug, and never let go. Not because *they* need it, but because *you* need to.

—Dr. Robert Sears, pediatrician,
author of *The Autism Book* and *The Vaccine Book*

INTRODUCTION

There is a revolution taking place, and it is happening now. Autism is a tragedy that shows up in households across America and around the world. As it takes root and grows in a generation of children, there is a resistance . . . a movement to take back our children from the world of autism and into a future full of hope.

The revolution is made up of parents who are armed with research papers, doctors who care about underlying medical conditions, and Google. They are fighting back against autism and the medical establishment that stood by while children faded away. It is a revolution fueled by love, hope, friendship, and determination. A change is coming, and parents are leading the way.

We, the moms and dad that you will meet in the pages of this book, started our parenting journey the way most do: filled with hopes and dreams for our children and the new life ahead of us. In each story, you will see that these dreams changed as the reality of speech delays, motor planning difficulties, mitochondrial dysfunction, gut dysbiosis, and a myriad of other health problems surfaced in our children. Our children are sick and need help. We are fighting to make them well, and we need doctors who can provide us with the tools necessary to treat these ailments.

All families facing autism need support, and we have found it in each other. Thanks to the modern world of social networking, a group of biomedical moms and a medically minded dad found each other and started talking. It began as a small group of people whose children were seeing the same homeopath, but it quickly transformed. The forum changed, other friends were added, and the group of strangers who once talked about homeopathic remedies became family. We had a lot of fun during our Facebook exchanges, and we discovered that we have some pretty hilarious members in our group, including a very talented individual who dubbed each of us with a creative nickname. You will see those nicknames used in our chapter titles. Many of our discussions still revolve around biomedical treatments, therapies, and autism interventions, but just as many are simply conversations that close friends have. Many of us have met in person at autism conventions, for a quick hello if we are traveling, or for a planned day of fun. We all genuinely like each other and are no longer in it just for the autism knowledge and pooled resources. We laugh together and cry together. When one of us hits a rough patch, the rest are there to offer support. When one of our children masters tying his shoe or riding her bike, we all break out the champagne.

We are a diverse group from the United States and abroad. We represent a myriad of religions and nationalities. Some of us speak different languages. Most of us now know more ways to curse in French than we ever thought we would! The reality is that our lives share one common denominator, a tie that binds. We are all working to take our children back from autism, ADHD, apraxia, sensory disorders, and mitochondrial dysfunction. One day, we all hope the tie that binds us together is a new reality: recovery. Some of us are there already.

We share our stories with you for a reason. This is a book we wish we could have read years ago. If you are new to the autism journey, we hope that you will learn from our friendships and from our experience. Find a support group or make your own if there isn't one around. The best thing you can do for yourself is to find like-minded people to share this journey with. If you are not living with autism, we hope that you will never join our ranks. Learn from our mistakes. Listen to what we have to say, and please, educate yourself when it comes to your children's health. We all dutifully listened to our physicians, and they came up short for our children with lasting consequences. Your children need you to be judicious about everything that is put into their bodies. Examine the ingredients in the foods they eat, give them pure drinking water, keep the toxic chemicals out of household cleaners, and read your vaccine inserts so you know what is going into them. The Thinking Moms' Revolution is about taking back the health of our children whether they have autism, asthma, sensory processing problems, or any of the other disorders that are found so frequently in our children today. We ask that as you read the pages of this book you do one very important thing. Think.

THE THINKING MOMS' REVOLUTION

TWONK: INTO THE FIRE

Oh, my good Lord! This is so *hard*! "Write it all down in a chapter," she said. "People need to know," she said. Love you, Goddess, but did I ever mention that I am the least creative lump of cellulite you could ever wish to meet? There are gluten-free muffins with more imagination than I've got. I've typed this out over a dozen times already. I've edited bits, added bits, stolen from the other girls. It's still not newsworthy. I've tried writing it from the child's point of view, my best friend's point of view, even the milkman's point of view (he lost a very profitable yoghurt order when we left, dontcha know), and still I'm coming up blank. The problem is I'm so damned English. My self-conscious British stiff upper lip keeps screaming in my head, *"You can't write that!"* Not that I'm inappropriate or anything. Much.

So I reckon the best way to get this over and done with is to imagine that I'm telling it to the girls. You know, the ones in the group. Because without them, I might very well still be convinced that there is no one else in the world quite like me and my kids. We were the outcasts forced to live on the edge of society because a mad old mum wouldn't accept what the doctors were saying. Don't get me wrong, we still are. The difference now is I know there are thousands of other people out here on the edge too, and we're all shouting the same thing.

"The vaccines did it!"

There . . . I feel better already.

Deep breath. *It's just like chatting waffle with the girls in a thread, that's all. No big deal. Right, here we go . . .*

The first thing I want to make absolutely clear is that what happened didn't happen to me. It happened to my children, and to my youngest son in particular. I am not a victim of autism, despite the fact my life has been forever changed by it. There have been sacrifices, and I consider those things to be casualties of autism: things like home, family, friends. Nothing major, right? But the only true victims here are the children. The rest of us, the parents, the siblings, the grandparents and teachers, we all need to think of ourselves as champions of autism, not victims, because without us, nothing will ever change, and the possibility that this travesty might go on indefinitely is simply not an option.

All four of my British-born kids carry labels. I actually like to think of them as designer kids because they have so many labels. The oldest was mostly nonverbal until the age of five, and now, at age eighteen, is officially labeled ADD (she's too lazy to be hyperactive) and LD (learning disabled) in math. When I was a kid, we used to call this phenomenon "crap at maths," but apparently now it warrants a clinical diagnosis. My eleven-year-old son is labeled ADHD with tendencies toward Asperger's syndrome. He's kind of like Rainman, except with this wonderfully wicked sense of humour. He scored 97 percent on his Iowa tests in third grade and frequently receives love letters from some of the most prestigious colleges in the USA. The problem is his sense of humour tends to be pretty highbrow and, therefore, flies over the heads of his classmates. Personally, nothing cracks me up quite like an algebra joke (yawn). Finally, the twins: Both boys, they're currently nine years old and separated by seventeen minutes. Twin One has congenital aortic stenosis and carries a diagnosis of autism and ADHD. He's very high functioning and should lose his autism diagnosis soon. He attends mainstream school, socializes well, has a few residual speech issues, but is, to all intents and purposes, almost fully recovered. Twin Two . . . well, this is really his story, and I have to write it down because he can't tell it himself.

My twins have always been opposites. Twin Two was always so happy, smiling, and flirting with anyone who caught his eye. He was the bigger of the two boys and immediately formed a connection with his twin brother. If Twin One was removed from the crib, Twin Two would instantly wake and start to cry. It was so cute that we used to do it purposely, just to say, "Awwwwwww." Twin One was the most miserable baby, always crying and throwing temper tantrums. By the time he was six weeks old, I was ready to trade him in for a newer model. I even commented about it to the doctor at their six-week well-baby visit. That's when the doctor pulled out his stethoscope and called the ambulance, and Twin One was diagnosed with severe aortic stenosis. Because of the heart defect, I paid extraspecial attention to the vaccine controversy happening in the media at the time. Some Hooray Henry doctor was being slagged off in the news again for suggesting a possible link between the MMR vaccine and sick kids. I didn't know all the details, but it made me ask the pediatrician what she thought was best. I asked her opinion, as if it would be unbiased, independent, based on real scientific evidence, and in the best interests of the child she was treating. She thought being vaccinated was best, and I now know that I should never have expected her to say anything different. She was a part of a machine—a cold-hearted, narrow-minded, bought-and-paid-for medical establishment—and she didn't even know it. But, based on the advice of this assumed superior intellect, I obediently led my lambs to the slaughter.

The boys started to get sick a lot: bronchiolitis, oral thrush, ear infections, random skin rashes, diarrhea, constipation, vomiting. It seemed as though every other week I found myself in the ER or the doctor's office. I didn't make a connection. My two older children were fully vaccinated and had had similar illnesses in their first year, especially my daughter. So, as far as I was concerned, it was all pretty much normal. (Earlier I mentioned that my daughter didn't start speaking fluently until she was five years old. I've no doubt anyone reading this would think I should have been alarmed by her lack of communication skills, and you're right. However, during the first five years of her life, she was dragged all over the world on irresponsible adventures. She lived in West Africa and Central

Europe and had all the required vaccines: yellow fever, hepatitis A, typhoid. You name it, I had her vaccinated with it for her own safety. Really, it wasn't because I was completely stupid, it was to protect her. She could repeat simple phrases in French and Dutch. I thought she was a genius whose speech had been affected by my own inability to stay in one place. Turns out she was echolalic. Who knew?) Towards the end of 2003, I received a letter from the local health authority advising me that all children born between 2000 and 2002 had been vaccinated with a dodgy batch of DTAP and meningitis C, and required unscheduled boosters.

We, the sheeple, would hereby like to confess: I never questioned a damn thing I was told to do. I simply went to extraordinary lengths—we were practically banned from attending baby clinic altogether, having been labeled a fire hazard—to have all three of my boys stuck with another round of unnecessary, unproven, unhealthy toxins in the ignorant belief that I was doing "the right thing."

The devastation was immediate. My youngest son developed a rash all over his body and ended up in the hospital yet again. He was found to be severely neutropenic and was treated with IV antibiotics to bring up his white blood cell count. It was probably the worst thing the ER doctors could have done. The antibiotics bound with the metals in the shots and carried them deep into the soft tissue of his organs, crossing the blood-brain barrier. He started to regress developmentally as he withdrew into his own world. Within the space of a few weeks, he lost most of his forty words, stopped making eye contact, stopped playing and laughing with his twin, developed a fascination with spinning objects, lost interest in the world around him, developed uncontrollable drooling.

You know the routine.

As much as I love the U.K., I have to say, hand on heart, that the way people there deal with mental disability is . . . well, pretty crap, really. It took five months for the appointment with a developmental pediatrician to come through.

Diagnosis: severe autism. ("He was born with it; you must have missed the signs. Don't let him set fire to himself until we can institutionalise him.")

I hung around with him for a while, thinking there would be a treatment, a therapy, something to pull him back from the edge of the abyss I was watching him slide into. There wasn't. I practically sold my soul to the pediatrician, begging her to do something about his constant fevers, diarrhea, constipation, yeast and bacterial infections. I even paid her in her private practice to bring the appointments forward as needed. A state-appointed early intervention speech therapist left her fingerprints in his arm when he wouldn't brush Barbie's hair. And so in 2005 I moved my family to the USA.

America . . . Where to start without offending anyone? OK, America, you can't go calling food things like chuck, grits, and Manwich and expect people to put it in their mouths. Pot stickers? Yuck! And why is there no news in your news programmes? I've learned more about side effects from pharmaceutical ads in the past six years than I've learned about world affairs from the news. Actually, the pharma ad thing is not a joke. I've been blown away by the in-your-face manipulation of everyday symptoms designed to convince an ever-paranoid population that they need to take a combination of pills every day for the rest of their lives in order to be healthy.

"Do you need to go to the bathroom when you leave the house? Ask your doctor if you have overactive bladder! (Possible side effects include nausea, dry mouth, and sudden death.)"

Did you know that some of the possible side effects for restless leg syndrome medication include uncontrollable gambling and sexual urges? No wonder the U.K. doesn't allow this kind of pharma advertising. If the British population were aware of this, there'd be a run on the National Health Service as millions of working-class numpties descended upon their GPs' offices doing their best interpretation of River Dance. The major thing America has going for it, and my reason for moving here in the first place, is simple: in the land of the free, nothing is free, but you can buy just about anything.

I bought a house, a car, a doctor, some hyperbaric chamber therapy, homeopathy, a Son-Rise start-up course, gluten/casein-free foods, private schooling, Applied Behavior Analysis (ABA), speech therapy, occupational therapy, chelation therapy, a whole array of prescription medicines, and enough biomedical interventions to revitalise a small country.

And the question on everyone's lips is, "How is he doing?"

My son has suffered two further regressions since arriving in America. Both times he tested positive for lead. Both times he was enrolled in the autistic unit of a local elementary school. Tests found the lead to be in painted furniture, which a teacher had allowed my son to repeatedly lick, despite a psychologist's report indicating pica to be a major concern. After two years of an intense ABA-based homeschool programme, he is beginning to vocalise once again. He can use the bathroom with assistance. He suffers with full-body dyspraxia and requires 24-hour care and supervision. He is currently under observation for seizure activity. In short, despite having made major gains in the past two years, my son is worse now than he was when we arrived.

America has been an incredibly bittersweet experience in so many ways. The hope we had when we came here, the relief experienced when a real medical doctor believed my son was physically ill, the expectations of starting each new protocol and treatment programme—all these things kept me on a path of determination to do as much as was humanly possible to improve my son's quality of life. As each of the other children was picked off with a label, and my youngest hit wall after wall, I found myself sitting alone at the PC into the small hours, researching every new treatment, every new fad. I rarely ventured out into the local community, instead surrounding myself and my children with therapists, doctors, teachers, and the odd autism parent rather than spending a lifetime repeating, "I'm sorry he put his hand in your food, he has autism" or "No, he isn't ill disciplined; he's going through a PANDAS flare."

It was a huge leap of faith into the misty depths of homeopathy that put me in touch with the group of people who were to become not only my support network but also my sanity. The group name has changed a few times, and good people have come and gone, but the die-hard queens (and king) of our group have remained constant and true to their cause. I'm not sure if our group dynamic is unique. I hope not—for the sake of all autism parents everywhere. Everyone should have a support group like ours. It's the first place I go when I have a question. They're the first people I share good news with, and I have learned so much because they have allowed me to share their autism lives. I had the great pleasure of meeting many of them last year at the AutismOne conference and had the weirdest experience of greeting old friends for the first time. As I sat amongst my family of strangers, I heard Alison McNeil say, "It's the other parents who will get you through."

And they do.

Bytes from the Count

I'm an engineer, specifically more of a computer hacker type. Got an obscure problem? Need an innovative solution? That's my specialty. A friend asked me to help with a problem at work and was marveling that I was able to fix her problem without knowing or understanding how her overall system worked. I told her that's the problem . . . you can't sit back and take the time to understand how the whole thing works. A good hacker dives in and zones in on what needs to be fixed. Usually, the fix needed is not the obvious fix. Out of the box thinking is standard matter of course here.

Sometimes I think docs and scientists sit there and overanalyze the problem . . . develop theories, test cases, conduct clinical trials . . . like I said, trying to understand the overall problem. Screw all that. I have one kid that needs to be fixed. And I'm on my quest for the ultimate hack. The autism hack.

MONEY'S TWO CENTS

Autism: the word that turns your world on its ear in less than thirty seconds flat. Autism: the word that causes your emotional state to deteriorate faster than you can say the word "insanity." Autism: the word that rips marriages apart, bankrupts your 401(k), and steals your plans and shreds them. Autism: I say it like it's a bad thing. Maybe it's not. Am I crazy? Well, there is probably an argument to be made for that, but hear me out.

Do I want my child to have autism? A very emphatic hell no! Can I change it? Sure I can! I really do believe that, and I am doing all I can to make sure that autism is history in our family. As much as I have prayed for the neurotypical fairy to visit my house overnight and make it all go away, that has not happened yet. Just for the record, it's not for lack of praying on my part either. As much as I want autism to take its rightful place in history, right this very second it has not done that. I am left to persevere. What is a person to do, you ask? Learn—a lot. Grow—more than you ever thought possible. Fight—harder than you ever thought you could. Love—with every cell of your being, and never waiver in your determination.

Autism has brought a lot of tears, fear, and anxiety into my life, but it has also brought wisdom, friends, support, and love. It has sent me on a journey that has taught me volumes, and I continue to learn daily. My life before autism had far more than its fair share of adversity and challenges. I am no stranger to struggle. In fact, there were so many difficult points in my life that after surviving it all,

I thought for sure I was "home free" and could bask in beautiful, relaxed glory as I sailed smoothly through the rest of my life. I figured that would only be fair. If wisdom comes through adversity, trust me, I'm a sage.

Realistically, I knew my daughter had autism before we even got the diagnosis. It was a bit odd, really. The sentence "She has autism" started popping into my head out of the blue when she was about fifteen months old. She would run endlessly back and forth in a line, much like the Energizer bunny on the television commercials. The sentence "She has autism" would appear as I broke into a sweat while chasing her madly around the playground ensuring her safety, while other mothers sat together casually chatting. The sentence was there when her beautiful babble descended into silence and morphed into a low guttural hum. Getting the diagnosis, for us, was more of a formality. My mommy gut knew, and my mommy gut did not want it to be true. I wished so badly that she would not have autism. In fact, I wished so hard it hurt.

Before my daughter was diagnosed, I scoured the Internet, searching for answers. I looked up her humming, lack of speech, and running around the house with some object clutched tightly in her fists to see what, if anything, it might mean. She did not play with toys in any conventional sense of the word "play." She would bang or drop them, but she did not play. It seemed to me that someone else out there must have dealt with something similar. I discovered that some had. Their children all had autism. I remember going to the First Signs website and watching videos. I remember bursting into tears as I watched other children behaving just as my sweet little girl did. They were all later diagnosed with autism. As I researched autism, I learned about Floortime, ABA, and biomedical therapies. I remember thinking, *Well, that's what we'll do then, if it really is autism (everyone is entitled to some denial, after all). We'll do biomed and Floortime.* I kept running across information about biomed therapy and having that same thought. It was almost as if the thought was not originating from within me. Similar to the sentence "She has autism" that kept springing into my head, this resolve to do biomed treatment and Floortime kept unexpectedly appearing.

In retrospect, I think the universe was very clearly saying, "Yo! Money! Wake up! Your kid has autism. Start with biomed treatment and Floortime. Get moving!" While that is exactly what happened, I have to admit it took me a lot longer than it should have. I lost a good year to my denial and waiting for an "official diagnosis" before I got a real move on it. That is one thing I do regret. The fact that she made good eye contact and had decent social referencing held up the formal diagnosis for more than ten months, and even then I had to directly ask for it. Developmental language delay, fine motor skill delay, play skill delay, and sensory integration disorder all added up to autism. Let's call it what it is so she can receive the services she needs. When the official diagnosis came, I remember thinking, *Autism? After all I've been through? Autism? Really?* I suppose this is where my previous experience with adversity came in handy. I didn't let myself get stuck there; I just rolled up my sleeves and dove right into the business of healing her.

As time goes on, I am getting much better at listening to my inner guidance. Take homeopathy, for example. It has been a big intervention for my daughter. I knew it would be important long before we started it. I read about author Amy Lansky's son's recovery on the web and got immediate goose bumps. I devoured her book *The Impossible Cure.* I had this deep inner knowing that homeopathy was one key to solving my daughter's puzzle. The time it took to get started with it was not simply due to my being slow or in denial. It was a matter of finding the right practitioner who could treat autism and all the complicated medical issues that go right along with it. I live in the sticks. We don't have many homeopaths around here, and I had no idea how to find a good one. I emailed Amy to see if she knew anyone in my area, and although she gave me a suggestion, it did not "feel right" to me. I knew my intuition would tell me when I found the right person. That took one full year. I knew I had found the right person when I got goose bumps again . . . and when I called to find about the waiting list it turned out there was a cancellation only two days later. Inner guidance and confirmation: beautiful synchronicity. I love it when that happens! It took about four months of doing homeopathy before we began seeing enormous gains. Homeopathy brought speech, receptive language, cognitive gains, and increased awareness. The best part was that, for my daughter, it did not come with regressions. Homeopathy is so gentle and easy. It is by far my favorite intervention to date.

I should probably stop momentarily to mention that I am obsessed with my daughter's recovery. The only time I am thinking of something else is when I am working with a client. Otherwise, every waking moment I think about her: what is happening in the moment, why it is happening, what needs to be done to make it better or boost the progress, where we go next and why. I am constantly researching, reading, networking, looking, hoping, praying, listening, loving, and believing. In the beginning, it was incredibly overwhelming. There are so many options and avenues to potentially pursue. Many are expensive and not covered by insurance. I wished with every cell of my being that I could somehow absorb all that I needed to know through osmosis. I felt this intense pressure about time. I feared that by the time I learned what I needed to know, I would miss the big window of opportunity where brain plasticity is most optimal. You always hear, "before age five." I remember looking at the voluminous stack of books and research thinking, *She's two. That's not a lot of time, and we have such a long way to go!* Now I am less concerned with time. I understand that there is no elusive door that closes at age five, and there are many treatment options that work very well beyond that age. Fear was an unwelcome resident that was quite challenging to evict in the early days, but it is important to evict it nonetheless. It is nothing but a barrier. The idea is to focus on what you have to do, where you need to go, and the concrete steps you need to take to get there. It is important to know that much like a standard GPS device, you will recalculate your journey many times.

Perseverance is important on this bumpy road. This is probably where my being obsessed with her recovery comes in handy. One can never know enough in order to heal a child: there is just so much to learn. I read books, blogs, magazine articles, research studies, message boards. I read and read and read and read some more. I try what makes sense to me and what my inner guidance leads me to. We have used many interventions: biomed, mHBOT, home-opathy, Floortime, and various types of energy healing, to name just a few. There is so much to learn, so much to do. I need a day with more hours in it. I used to think I was busy before autism. The fact that I thought that amuses me. I was simply delusional back then. *Now* I'm busy.

I should probably pause to mention that many strange things happen on this road to healing autism. Your child progresses and regresses and progresses again. Regressions frustrate you; progressions delight you. You learn a lot about poop. Yes, you read that correctly; I said you learn a lot about poop. If people had told me years ago that I would know this much about poop, I would have thought they were crazy. Why would anyone need to know so much about poop? But it's true: autism parents talk a lot about poop. Sometimes they even post pictures about poop. In fact, I believe there is a whole entire blog dedicated to poop. Poop, as it turns out, can tell you a great deal about what is going on in a body and what you need to do to heal it. For example, fluffy, airy poop means that there is yeast overgrowth. Sticky poop also means that there is yeast overgrowth. Sandy poop indicates an oxalate problem. Black specks in poop indicate die-off. Green poop is evidence of bacteria. See? Look at how much you just learned about poop! These poop inspections bring mixed feelings: "Oh *no*, there is a problem. But oh *yay*, I can do something about it! Afterwards, I will see more progress, and she will feel better!" There is nothing more thrilling than seeing your child respond positively to an intervention. Excitement pulses through my veins as I witness her becoming healthier and returning to us.

You learn about a lot of things on this road. You learn about viruses, yeast, bacteria, neurological conditions, mitochondrial dis-orders, metabolic disorders, allergies, intolerances, mast cells, gas-trointestinal disorders, and much, much more. Most autism parents discover early on that they know more about autism and treating it than their pediatricians do. While that can be uncomfortable, the really good pediatricians learn from you and go on to help other patients heal and thrive. It is a beautiful domino effect of healing. Doctors who balk and ridicule you are nothing more than barriers to healing. Thank them for their time, and move on. As a parent of a child on the spectrum, you learn very quickly to advocate for your child. Do what works, and leave what does not, including doctors.

Most parents of children with autism should be awarded honorary MDs. It is a bit amusing, really. Our medical vocabulary is expansive and an integral part of our daily life. That can sometimes make us difficult to understand. I realized this one day while giving my mother-in-law an update. I was undeniably speaking a foreign language as I briefed her on cerebral folate deficiency and how a dairy-free diet can down-regulate folate receptor autoimmunity. It amuses me that I did not even like science in school, and yet today I live immersed in it. I'm okay with that. You do what you need to do to heal your child. You smile, you cry, you pull your hair out, you hope, you dream, you try, you fall, you get up, and you try again. Most of all, you *know*. You must know with every fiber in your being that your child will recover. And you must never give up.

In addition to the practical knowledge I have learned about healing my daughter's body, autism has also brought an inordinate opportunity for me to examine my beliefs and attitudes and choose the ones that propel me and my family forward. I have a friend who spends a great deal of time being immobilized by her son's autism. Her son is three months younger than my daughter. Every day she looks at her son's baby pictures and cries. Every time I have gotten together with her, she says the same thing, "I look at all these typical kids, and then I look at my son and ask 'why'—of all kids, why him, why us?" My response has become predictable. I tell her it is okay to visit that place, but one cannot live there. Truth be told, I hate visiting that place. It is depressing, and it does nothing to heal my daughter. It also does absolutely nothing for my energy level. Who knows specifically why her son or my daughter is affected? Why me? Well, then again . . . why *not* me? Perhaps my child was chosen because I will be part of the ranks to search every corner of the universe for a way to heal her and others like her. Perhaps because I am someone who will not be bullied into silence and will fight hard for what is best for her. Perhaps because I will take an active part in finding a cure for autism and learning how to prevent it in the first place. Perhaps kids with autism are here to make us become responsible inhabitants on the earth. There are so many food allergies and chemical sensitivities that perhaps these kids are here to green the earth and bring us back to responsible, sustainable living. Yes, it's true. I tend to look for the bigger spiritual answers. Who knows what specifically makes one child vulnerable and not another? One thing is for sure: autism statistics are on the rise, and it is terrifying. Something must be done.

I have come to realize that there will always be two perspectives: a positive one and a negative one. You can consciously choose to be in one or the other. For me, this road needs to be positive. My daughter deserves that, and I deserve that. I have been blessed with a very happy, beautiful little girl whose smile melts my heart and whose laughter makes my spirit soar. She has an impish sense of humor and loves to surprise you. I don't want to miss a second of her due to worry, negativity, or fear. Nor do I want her to sense the negativity and believe that it is somehow about her as a person. She is nothing short of amazing. She has blessed my world, and I feel honored to be her mother. I believe and know, with the deepest sense of knowing there is, that she will be okay. I know that I am being guided to take the next right step for her. I may flounder from time to time, but the guidance always comes. I need only to pause and listen to the wise whispering within. Anxiety and panic drown out sage intuition. Choosing not to participate in chaos quiets the fear and allows me to know what to do next. Trusting that is key.

I am learning to keep positive people in my life and limit the time I spend with people who are negative. I cannot afford to give any of my energy to negativity. I cannot afford to waste a moment to doubt or fear. Fear, after all, is only false evidence appearing real. My daughter's recovery and well-being are too important, and so are my own health and well-being. I read something each day that empowers and grounds me in a peaceful place. Whether it is an excerpt from Don Miguel Ruiz's *The Four Agreements* or Barry Neil Kaufman's *Happiness Is a Choice*, I make sure to read something affirming, even if it is two in the morning. It makes an enormous difference in the quality of my life. Even now, as I write, I can sense the difference. Naming off the various problems I am working to solve as I weave through the maze of recovering my daughter sends tension through my shoulders and stomach. Focusing on choosing happiness, making empowered decisions, and trusting in divine guidance leaves me feeling peaceful and focused. It is important to stay in today. It is the only point of power we really have. Giving our energy to positive efforts manifests a positive, happy future. It is simple quantum physics: like energy attracts like energy. Take the next right step for your child, and trust it while making sure to enjoy the moment.

Putting this into practice is really not all that difficult. Consciously choosing to underscore the positive makes such a difference. My daughter recently went through a sizeable regression. We were treating her for cerebral folate deficiency. After an amazing initial two weeks, it all crashed headlong into disaster. Nothing seemed to be working to turn it around. It would be easy to feel discouraged in this situation. In the midst of this regression, I opted to highlight the good things: she was progressing in her play; she was feeding her baby dolls and lovingly putting them to bed; she was putting her "little people" down the slide while gleefully exclaiming, "Weeee!" At the end of that day, I felt so much better that I had reveled in the positive while acknowledging the challenges rather than vice versa. Sharing that with people who understand gave me an additional boost.

In the beginning, this road felt very lonely. My friends all had typical kids and really had no frame of reference for understanding the path I was on. The couple of local people I met who had kids on the spectrum were so overwhelmed by it that they could barely move. I turned to the Internet. The Internet connected me with some incredible people. There are many forums out there that will assist you in healing your child. I found that some of the forums are fraught with insults and arguments as some people have trouble believing that there is more than one trail to the top of the mountain. I limit my time in such places. Essentially, I started out on some Yahoo! groups, found another message board or two, and ultimately landed on Facebook. I connected with a group of people using classical homeopathy to heal autism. We shared our stories and problem-solved together. Eventually, a fairly sizeable group of us realized that we needed to be creative and combine many therapies in order to fully heal our children. Thus, The Thinking Moms' Revolution was born. "TMR," as we call ourselves, came together to share our knowledge of biomed, homeopathy, energy medicine, conventional therapies, and pretty much anything and everything that we had knowledge of. We have talked about camel milk, goat yogurt, kefir water, Mito cocktails, BioSet, CEASE, homeopathy, doctors, lawyers, schools, Son-Rise, ABA, speech therapy, MRIs, probiotics, enzymes, and of course, poop. There is something so special about this group of people and the collective wisdom and compassion we share. Becoming part of this extraordinary group was the first time I ever felt truly at home on this journey.

TMR is an exceptional, uplifting group. It does not matter if it is one in the morning or one in the afternoon, there is a Thinking Mom (or Dad) there ready to help. If you need emotional support, problem solving, opinions, marriage counseling (yes, I got some), or supplement help, you will find it with them. I had traveled this road for a long time very much alone, and although I did not mind that, it was a pretty lonely journey. My friends did not understand what my life was like, how exhausting it can get, or what I do. They could not understand why it was not possible for me to spontaneously take my child to a park in the middle of a noisy city and then eat at any old place. Sensory issues and special diets confound them. The idea that it is impossible to predict whether my child will have a stellar or disastrous day eludes them. Making plans with friends became impossible. Because of that, you can lose friends on this road. People who are not on this path really do not understand the energy and effort it takes to heal a child on the spectrum. To be sure, the friendship losses are sad. But I am gaining a healthy little girl who is coming back to me, and along the way I am gaining many beautiful friends. TMR members understand it all: no explanation needed.

The first real-life TMR-fest occurred at AutismOne in Chicago in 2011. Although I was unable to attend in person, I was online every night, reading the details. Twonk took great notes and posted them as a document so that all the Thinking Moms could benefit from the lectures, regardless of whether we were there in person or not. They posted pictures of their first embraces, their first meal together, and their pictures with autism healer celebrities. It was almost as if we were all there together.

The most amazing experience I had was a mini TMR-fest in my own home. Sunshine was driving quite a distance to bring her son to a specialist in the area. Those of us who lived in the greater vicinity jumped on the opportunity to get together. We chose my house as the location because it has an in-ground swimming pool, fenced-in yard, and sensory room in the basement: all helpful things for kids on the spectrum. We started planning for it a month in advance. Lo and behold, although we had been having a beautiful, dry, sunny summer, it was raining that day. Autism moms are flexible. We swam in the rain; you get wet swimming anyway! Many kids on the spectrum love the pressure of the water on their bodies. It can be so soothing for them. We all laughed and played together. The day may have been raining and gray, but the sun was shining brightly in our hearts. As I sat on the floor in my living room, holding my napping daughter, I glanced around at the children playing and laughing. I heard a conversation about biomed taking place over organic guacamole and tortilla chips in the kitchen. I closed my eyes for just a moment and felt the most incredible feeling of connected peace sweep over me. What a gift! Everyone was comfortable, happy, and at ease. No one had to worry about "what her child might do," because whatever that child did was just fine with all of us. We talked about mitochondrial cocktails, homeopathy, chelation, CEASE, and speech. We discussed coping, energy levels, progress, and triumphs. We supported each other and loved each other. The feeling of camaraderie was unparalleled and so fulfilling. How I had missed this! How happy I am that we have found each other!

It does not matter what is happening, this beautiful group of people will be there. Having a bad day? Talk to them about it. Have a problem you cannot figure out? Post about it, someone will have a good idea. When one of us is down, we are always signing on to see how that person is doing. We make it a point to check in on that person and offer support. These people have become my trusted, beloved friends who understand me, my family, and my life. These are people who care with all their being. These are people who breathe life back into me after the day has sucked it all out, and I hope I do the same for them. Need to know about juicing? Tex is your woman. Want to know about Andy Cutler's chelation? Sugah is your girl. Want to know about stem cells, adrenal glands, IVs, and just so happen to need a good laugh? The Count is your man. Need information on Son-Rise? Ask Princess. Want to learn about LEAP? Talk with Mama Mac. There are twenty-three Thinking Moms and one Dad in total. We laugh, cry, and celebrate together. I do not know where I would be without them, and I am really glad that I do not have to find out.

It is quite a journey. If you are on this journey, remember a few important things: Highlight the positive, evict fear and listen to your heart, be present in the moment, take the next right step, and find some good friends to connect with. Trust your gut. Rest assured that while I am waiting for The Count to come up with the ultimate autism hack, I will be doing the very same.

Poppy Flips Autism the Bird

There are three things that can't be long hidden:
the sun, the moon, and the truth.
—BUDDHA

It was August 2003. I sat on the edge of the tub in my tiny, one-bedroom apartment and stared at that pee stick for what seemed like hours. I was terrified. How could I be someone's mother? I can't keep plants alive, and I gag at the sight of dog crap! I never really thought about having kids. I was terrified but in love already. I knew his name right away. I knew I was having a boy; perhaps I willed it. I would make this work.

Thankfully, I had a good job with great medical benefits when I got pregnant. I found a good OB/GYN right away and made my first appointment. I remember sitting in the waiting room, going through the pages and pages of new-patient intake forms, and answering questions about everything under the sun. I checked the "other" box and filled in the blank: "I have two twin cousins on my mother's side who have autism." You see, autism first came into my life a long time ago when it was still this rare enigma of a psychiatric disorder. The shift in causation theories was just turning from the cold "refrigerator mother" theory to the theory of bad genes. It wrecked my family's world back then, but that's a story for another time. Let's just say I was well aware of autism from the start.

During my pregnancy, I craved sautéed spinach and garlic and would eat entire pints of grape tomatoes in a clip. Morning sickness was minimal, and overall I felt better than I had ever felt. I took my prenatal vitamins and never missed a doctor's appointment. I was so excited to start this chapter of my life. When I started to look into pediatricians, I decided on one who was recommended to us. There are a lot of things I'd like to call him, but I'll try to keep it clean and just use Dr. Soprano. Slicked back hair, Cuban shirt . . . the whole nine. But I liked him. I trusted him. I decided he would be the guy.

April 2004. The big day came. I checked into the hospital at 8:00 a.m. to bring my sweet boy into the world. I was completely unprepared for what was about to ensue. I was going to be induced. No big deal at all. They do it all the time! Trust the doctors . . . they know what they are doing, right? The nurses struggled with the IV, leaving both my arms bloody and feeling like chopped meat. They finally had to use a vein in my hand and got the Pitocin drip started to induce labor. Then the pain came. Like a freight train. Like nothing I had ever imagined it could be. They also loaded me up with antibiotics because I was a strep B carrier. Again, just routine procedures for cases like these. Not to worry.

"Here, honey, let us give you a little something for the pain. We use it all the time." Stadol. An opiate. Yeah, I wish I knew then what I know now. It put me on my ass! I was so out of it that I would pass out in between contractions. This went on for hours. At midnight, my OB came in and said they were giving me another dose of Stadol to get me through the night. If I hadn't given birth by morning, we would have to do a C-section. Trust the doctor. I look back, and it makes me sick to think of the toxic soup my poor baby was swimming in.

Within a half hour, I was fully dilated. My body was ready to rock and roll, but my brain was drowning in opiates. I don't remember most of the delivery. It consisted of pushing and nodding out. It was a horrible experience. I was completely out of control of my own body for the birth of my first child. But *finally*, he was here. It was like the moment they cut the cord I came out of the fog. The nurse handed me this little creature wrapped up like a glowworm, and I saw this perfect little face. My sweet baby boy. Sheer perfection. Within minutes, they swooped him away to the nursery and gave him his necessary shots. Trust the doctors. They know what they are doing.

I had already decided that I was going to bottle-feed. After all, I was bottle-fed. We were all bottle-fed. The doctor said it's just as good as breast milk. J took to the bottle, did his first poop, and was cleared to go home. I think back to those first few days home and curse my naivety. I was sitting on the couch with this little peanut. So new, so tiny, so wonderful. I gave him a bottle, and he chugged it like he had never eaten in his life. He was sucking so ferociously that the bottle actually made a pop sound when I pulled it from his mouth. I sat him up a bit and rubbed his little back for a burp. He let one rip . . . followed by a stream of projectile vomit that could fill buckets. *Holy shit!* I sat there stunned and in shock. I had never seen anything like this before. He didn't cry or make a peep, and actually looked relieved and relaxed. I called the doctor immediately. He said it was just a dairy intolerance and advised me to just switch to soy formula. This type of vomiting continued throughout his first year of life. But the doctor was not concerned . . . babies spit up. No big deal. Calm down, *mom*. Don't worry about it. J also began developing sores on his body that would go from a small hive to an open wound. One on his hand. Another on his ear. One on his thigh. Each time, off to the doctor we went. Here, just put this cream on it and give him some antibiotics. It's nothing to worry about.

This scene played out numerous times. We were at the doctor's constantly for colds, coughs, or sores, and each time we left with a prescription for antibiotics. A few times we got a bonus deal and left with our scheduled vaccinations. Must keep on the sacred schedule! And let's not forget the poop. It was (and is to this day) of a foul, yellow, soft-serve consistency. Frequent and abundant. Again, don't worry. Babies poop. Other than this, J was perfect. He hit all his milestones on time. He slept through the night. He was an easy baby. Very calm and mellow. He rarely cried. I thought I hit the baby jackpot! My house was cleaner than it ever was. This mommy stuff was a piece of cake!

In October 2005, I found out I was pregnant again. This pregnancy was much different. I was sick all the time. I had heartburn constantly and would puke from the smell of garbage on the street. I had such bad lower back pain I could barely walk. At the same time, we realized J was not talking like he should. Family tried to assure me. The firstborn always talks late, especially boys. Still, something told me I should worry. And boy, I was worried.

On our next "well-care" visit, I flat out asked Dr. Soprano, "Doc, I'm really worried that he isn't talking. Do you think he has autism?" He looked at me and smirked. Looking back, it was at that moment that he diagnosed me with NMS (neurotic mommy syndrome). "Look at this kid!" he replied. "Does he look at you? Does he hug and love you? Does he answer to his name? This kid doesn't have autism! Now here, hold his leg while we give him his shots." Phew! That's a load off my mind! If the doctor says J's fine, he must be fine, right?

The time came to check into the hospital for the arrival of the new guy. I learned my lesson last time and refused Stadol, but I was still induced with the Pitocin and given antibiotics for the strep B. I remember every moment of the delivery and was present in the experience. It was very different from the first go-around. When my second son arrived, I looked at his little face and thick dark hair and was in love all over again. O was here. I was so excited and anxious to get home so my big boy could finally meet his little brother. The reaction was not what I expected. J cried instantly at the sight of him. He gagged when O would drink from a bottle. He could barely stand to look at him, like the baby creeped him out. There was no bonding. No connection. This was way beyond an adjustment to a new sibling period. It broke my heart. J was supposed to be my little helper with this new baby, but he could barely stand to be in the same room as him. By the way, the words still were not coming like they should have. All he would say were numbers. He would read numbers off of everything, but that was it.

He's fine. Boys are late talkers. He's fine. Why does he keep banging his head? He's fine. He really loves lining up his cars. He's fine. The firstborn always starts late. He's fine. He's fine. He's fine. I kept telling myself this.

During this time, we relocated from a major metropolitan city to a rural mountain town to run a business. And when I say rural, I mean *rural*. Big mistake. Living in the boonies stuck in the house with two kids while neither of them is talking yet . . . I was freaking out. I figured J wasn't going to talk while he was stuck in the house with O and me, so I decided I would enroll him in the little pre-school in town. Some peer interaction and modeling should bring him right out of his shell. I expressed my concerns to the director, and she agreed that it would be good for him. She also assured me that the fact he wasn't potty trained yet wasn't an issue for enrollment. She asked that I bring him in and give it a try.

It was a few days before Halloween 2007. We snapped pictures, put his new backpack on, and headed to school. I felt so hopeful. This was going to be what he needed. He would be fine. Off he went. No problem. No protest. That's my boy; go with the flow. When I went to pick him up that afternoon, the director and the teacher asked if I had a minute to talk. I remember sitting at the small kid table across from them, saying, "You think something is wrong too, don't you?" They nodded, and the director said, "Yes, we do."

I remember that moment like it was yesterday. I got a wave of relief that I wasn't *crazy*, instantly followed by the feeling of being kicked in the gut and having the air knocked out of me. Fuck. I was right. Fuck. Now what?

I am forever grateful to those women though. Validation. They are the ones who got the ball rolling on assessments and therapies for J. They also agreed that O should be evaluated and got early intervention going for him. I owe them so much.

Frantic, I called my mother and brother. Until this point, they thought I was a bit crazy and worrying about nothing. When I told them what the director said and that we were going forward with evaluations, they were devastated. My brother sobbed. The next day, they were both at my doorstep. They rallied around me immediately and have never stopped. Without them, I'm not sure where we would be. My brother walked in and hugged me tighter than ever before. He said he was so sorry that he ever doubted me and would never question me again. He was so upset that I knew something was up and no one listened to me. This was Lesson #1 in autism. Trust your mommy gut. I would *never* doubt my mommy-gut again. Ever.

I started researching the Internet and devouring books. I couldn't believe what I was reading. A possible vaccine connection?? No one told me about a fucking vaccine connection! What do you mean there's fucking *mercury* in the shots? Not *once* since autism came into my family's life back in the '80s had I ever heard this! I kept reading. A book brought me through a full range of emotions: rage, sadness, guilt. I was a total mess. How the fuck could this happen in *America*? How could this happen to my baby?

I decided that the boys would get no more shots, but I felt so confused. I read about many of these children who had seizures. J never did. (In retrospect, he did in fact have petit mal seizures as a baby. He would tense up, open his mouth wide, and squeeze the rail of the crib. Of course, I told Dr. Soprano about it, and he said that J was just so excited and overstimulated. Now do you understand why I want to wring this idiot's neck? Trust the doctors.) I never saw a full-blown regression after shots. My J just slowed developmentally. How could this be? My head was spinning.

During this time, we began school therapy for J and home-based early intervention for O. The initial assessment process was heartbreaking. It was a surreal experience to sit there and have a stranger ask you questions about what your child could and couldn't do. It made the deficits a blaring reality. I realized that things were worse than I had thought. The speech therapist doing the evaluation for J suggested "The Diet" (an elimination of gluten, casein, and other food allergens common in kids with ASD). My eyes lit up! I told her I had been reading up on it. She gave me two books to read: *Special Diets for Special Kids*, by Lisa Lewis, and *Children with Starving Brains*, by Dr. Jacquelyn McCandless. I devoured them. Could it be that this was true— that diet could help eliminate some autistic symptoms—and this was a medical autoimmunity illness and not just a psychiatric disorder? Why was no one yelling about this from the rooftops? J was already limiting his food selection and eating only the Fab Five foods (chicken nuggets, fries, waffles, peanut butter sandwiches, and pizza). I decided to start the diet ASAP. Living where I did made it feel almost impossible to start. The stores were an hour away and didn't have a selection of specialty foods at all. I was overwhelmed. I wasn't seeing changes. My children were not eating. But, I kept it up for a few months.

It wasn't until April 28, 2008, that I finally had an appointment with a pediatric neurologist. My mom came up to go to the doctor with me. We loaded the kids in the car and jumped on the ferry across the lake to the Children's Hospital. It was a cold and rainy day. We sat quietly on the ride over, mentally preparing ourselves for what we knew was ahead. The doctor sat with us for quite some time, observing J and asking questions. Then she looked at me and said, "I believe your boy is on the spectrum. He has PDD-NOS." I knew it was coming, but I could have never prepared myself for that moment. I was numb. Secretly, I still hoped I was wrong and a little therapy would bring him up to speed. We sat on the ferry back home, and I mourned the loss of the dreams I had for my beautiful boy. I wanted to scream at the top of my lungs and smash shit. Inside, I was a complete mess but held it together for my mom and the kids. I had to be the strong one. I always am the strong one, after all.

I slipped into a *bad* depression for a few weeks, unable to sleep, crying constantly, having no appetite, losing weight, drinking more wine than I should have. I knew I had to pull myself out of it. I had to be strong for my babies. I knew I couldn't stay in the boonies anymore. My kids needed good doctors and services close to them, not an hour away. It was freezing cold, and they were sick all the time. I had developed a severe allergy to snow. I was completely over mountain living. We decided we would move to Florida. My mom had a place for us to stay until we got on our feet and could start fresh. Off we were again. I took charge and made arrangements for everything they would need. Florida would be good for us. Sun. Beach. Warmth. We needed a fresh start. In June 2008, we headed south.

I found my niche in Florida. I networked, met other mothers, and formed a few of the most important friendships in my life. I was involved and didn't feel so alone in this. On April 28, a year to the day after J's diagnosis, I finally got an appointment and took O for an official evaluation. The neurologist (another smug, useless professional) watched my little son run around. She asked about language, and I told her he had none. He would just scream and make a few sounds for things he wanted. After about ten minutes of more standard questions, she said, "He is PDD-NOS with ADHD and a mood disturbance. I will write you a prescription for Risperdal." Um, *excuse me*? He was three! I was not giving him Risperdal, a drug I was quite familiar with. I knew it had horrible side effects and was way overprescribed, especially to children. Thank you for your time. When I asked when she would write something up for me so that I had documentation of the diagnosis for services and planning, she took out a prescription pad, scribbled her diagnosis, and told me to come back in six months. Needless to say, we never went back.

I adjusted and was holding my own. My family and friends stuck by me. I knew we would be fine. It was through this network of moms that I heard about an upcoming autism conference held right in Florida. The organization sponsoring the conference, National Autism Association, was offering scholarships. I had never heard of them before but decided to apply for a scholarship and got one. Honestly, I was more looking forward to a weekend away by myself at a nice hotel than the conference. I booked a room and looked forward to a frosty drink by the pool, free of diapers, meltdowns, and Nick Jr. Two of my new friends were going too, so I was looking forward to getting some girl time. We all deserved the break. Little did I know that this would be the starting point on our road to recovery.

I got to the hotel, checked in for the conference, and made my way to the room. I dropped off my things, grabbed my notebook, and hit the lecture halls. I attended presentations on things I had never heard of given by doctors that packed the house. Numerous "standing room only" discussions on things like methylation, autoimmune disorders, IEPs, GFCF, IgG, HBOT, and MTHFR. It was like autism alphabet soup! My head was spinning. I saw charts, diagrams, and slides fitting for a med school presentation. As I sat in one lecture in particular, I remember feeling a headache coming on. I took off my glasses, rubbed my eyes, and looked around the packed room. It struck me that it was full of women with a few men peppered in. They looked tired and stressed as they scribbled down every word and made notes on diagrams in the presentation handouts. They carried binders full of assessments, lab results, and evaluations. These ladies were on a mission. I realized that I was not alone. There was an army of us.

I chatted with mothers from around the country about their children. We discussed symptoms, meltdown, obsessions, and poop. A lot of talk about the poop (Lesson #2 in autism—it always comes back to the poop). I sat and listened to one story after another about normal development, regression, medical illness, food allergies, as well as various interventions that helped. My head was spinning again. Everything I was ever taught to believe was going down the toilet fast. I learned that the doctors weren't always right. I learned that trusting your gut is crucial. I learned that vaccine injury is real. I learned that autism is, in fact, a vaccine injury. I learned that kids *can* and *do* get better! We drank wine, and I listened to one heartbreaking story after another about having sick children and being dismissed by the mainstream medical community. I felt so bad for these women. Then it hit me . . . I *was* one of these women. It was overwhelming. Off to bed . . . my head was going to explode.

I woke up the next morning feeling foggy. I'm sure the wine had a little something to do with it, but it was so much more than that. I made my way to get coffee to lift the fog and couldn't help but revisit my conversations from the night before. Could this really be happening? Was it possible that the medical establishment had dropped the ball? It was blowing my mind. I felt like I was on overload. I felt nauseous. I wanted to get home and hug my kids. I couldn't believe this was all happening. I felt like I was in a bad conspiracy theory movie.

Life hasn't been the same since then. I was full of hope, but I was also full of rage. I got home and instantly started the boys on a GFCF diet. Cold turkey. I also started with some melatonin I purchased there to help with sleep (until then, O slept for only a couple of hours at a time). This was the first night in a *long* time that he slept for more than three hours. I was thrilled! I spent hours and hours on the Internet, searching and reading scores of journal articles and special diet cookbooks. I was determined to get my children better. I marched into my new Florida pediatrician's office, handed her a list of labs I had from the presentations, and demanded we do some testing and get a referral to a GI doctor (who turned out to be yet *another* useless professional) for the boys. She said (and won my respect from this), "I don't know what any of these tests will show in relation to autism, but I will run what I can for you." Within a few months of the diet and supplementation, O went from no language to stringing three and four words together. *It was working!* We never looked back.

Through my new network of super moms in town, I found a doctor who took the boys' insurance and believed in biomedical treatments for many illnesses, not just autism. She worked in conjunction with a chiropractor, and she herself had a child with autism. I took my lab reports and went to the first appointment. By now, I had taken so much of the incredible information I obtained from the conference and various websites (TACA is *invaluable!*) and had my boys in full swing on the diet, and I was using probiotics, multivitamins, and fish oil. I had my notebook in hand, full of a list of things I wanted to talk with the doc about. I was a new kind of mother. No more blindly trusting the doctors.

We discussed the boys, their behaviors and GI issues. It was when I said, "What do you think of glutathione?" that I knew the conversation could have gone one of two ways. She could tell me to get off Google, or she could answer my question. She smiled and said, "I was *just* going to talk to you about glutathione!" I heard angels singing. She was a keeper! A doctor who *really* listened!

I kicked into biomedical treatments hard and started hemispheric integration, ABA therapy, and chiropractic adjustments. The boys were doing fantastic. Baby steps, but obviously my children were so much healthier than they had been. I began removing soy and oats from their diet and served only organic food. I eliminated as many toxins from their environment as I could and still do today. I kept my local health food store in business, but it was all worth it. I would sell my spare organs if it got me what my boys needed.

My free time (ha ha) is now spent at the computer, searching and devouring medical journals and information on treatments. Facebook is an integral part of my life. I have met hundreds of people going through the same things. I have found a group of women and men across the country on a mission to help their kids and to fight the injustices that have been done. Brilliant, tenacious, and driven folks who will go to the end of the Earth for their children. People I now consider my family. Thanks to Facebook, I can share in the joys and struggles of my brothers and sisters in this journey. I can get an answer to a question in seconds, complete with links to citations. I can rant. I can laugh. I can offer support and ideas. I can talk about poop in an open manner. I always say, "You don't really get it until you've got it." No one can truly understand what it's like to raise children with autism except other people who live it.

My boys are far from being recovered from autism, but I will continue to drive the recovery bus until the wheels fall off. We have come so far. Probiotics and good, clean, *real* foods are helping heal their guts. We are killing the parasites and yeast that riddle their systems. We are starting hyperbaric oxygen therapy to work on increasing blood flow and decreasing inflammation. Glutathione and detoxification supports are helping them rid their bodies of toxins. We also use homeopathy in a variety of ways. There are many things that can be done, and I'm willing to continue on this path until my boys have recovered.

We have an incredible network of incredible people in our lives. My two beautiful, sweet, funny boys love to play *together*, love their family and friends, and are getting healthier day by day. J loves swimming, music, and instruments, is fantastic at spelling, and loves the iPad. He has various medical issues and food sensitivities that we are addressing. He still really struggles with expressive and receptive language and motor skills. He can talk to me, and I understand him. He has work to do but is a long way from reciting numbers.

Then there's O. Ahhh, my little wild child! *Great* language, funny, sassy, loves Ozzy and old '80s metal (he is *sooo* my son). He loves *Star Wars*, Legos, and fighting with his big brother. *They* are the true heroes in this story.

I can't give up hope. Hope is all I have to fuel me. Don't get me wrong; I have my moments on the kitchen floor, covered with boogies from crying. It's hard. *Really* hard. But I wash my face and play through, just like everyone else. Equating it to the stress of soldiers in combat is so fitting. It's a constant battle. Doctors, insurance companies, politicians, school districts, the mainstream. I am not some wacko, tinfoil-hat-wearing mother looking for something to blame. I am an intelligent, educated, strong woman. I watched this all happen. I will continue to fight. I have to. I will fight for my kids, my friends, their children, and the children and families who will face autism in the future. I will fight for the doctors and researchers who are ridiculed and persecuted for going against the grain and really helping our kids. I will fight for healing. This is an epidemic of mass proportion. It's not going away. It's getting worse.

Autism has changed my perspective on so much—food, medicine, politics, big business, relationships, money, priorities. Everything changes. For the most part, things have changed for the better. I am smarter. I am stronger. I now *really* think for myself and follow my instincts. I have lifelong family to help me get through. I have the truth. Someday soon, the rest of the world will *listen* to the truth, too. We are getting there. People are waking up. Hopefully, our stories will help that along.

LOVE AND SAVAGE

My husband and I met in 1991, and it was love at first sight. Completely cliché, but he was my Prince Charming. We were only teenagers, but I knew we were going to get married and have kids. We both wanted a big family. I had visions of the big house in the suburbs, a white picket fence, a dog, a minivan, the whole nine yards. I was excited to be a soccer mom, and my husband was excited for his boys to play football just like he did. We were perfect for each other, and we were in love. We got married, and I was overjoyed when I became pregnant with our first child: a boy. Naturally, my husband was ecstatic. He had such plans for his first son and talked incessantly about the things they would do together and how he would share in his hopes and dreams. It was amazing to watch my husband grow more and more excited each day during my pregnancy. When I gave birth to our son, I was so proud to name him after his father. My husband didn't leave my side the entire time I was in the hospital. The joy on his face when he held his son was a moment I will never forget. We were living our dream, and at that moment I was foolish enough to think things were going to stay that way, absolutely perfect. But life had other plans for us. It seems like a lifetime ago since that day in the maternity wing of the hospital.

Michael got all of his shots on schedule, two months, four months, six months, nine months, and twelve months. Back in 2002, there wasn't a whole lot of information about autism and vaccine-related injury, but there was some. I was nervous about vaccinating. It always made me uneasy. I talked it over with my pediatrician, who assured me that I was doing the right thing by protecting my child. I was a loving mother who was making sure her child did not come down with a devastating illness. My sister's son was already exhibiting signs of autism, and it did worry me that there might be a genetic component and the vaccines would be too much for my little guy. I questioned the use of thimerosal and its neurotoxic potential, but I allowed myself to be swayed by the pediatrician that the minute amount in the vaccine couldn't possibly cause any problem. This is one time in my life when I should've listened to that voice of doubt in my head that something was not right. I didn't feel comfortable with vaccines. I wanted to know more, do more research, make sure they were safe, but I fell for the propaganda hook, line, and sinker. The pediatrician won out; my guilt won out. How could I refuse the shot and possibly leave my newborn baby at risk for a dreaded disease? I could never forgive myself if he got polio, measles, or hepatitis. The pediatrician made me feel as if these diseases were lurking around every corner, just waiting to invade my precious newborn child. Every well-child visit (ironic they are called "well-visits"), Michael received three or four vaccinations. After every round of shots, he would develop a fever of 102, sometimes 104, and every time I called the doctor in a panic. Every time, I was reassured that these "side effects" were normal and nothing to be concerned about. I was just being an overly anxious mother.

About the time my son was four months old, after a round of shots, reflux kicked into high gear. He started projectile-vomiting all over the place. After his six-month shots, he developed a huge swelling on his leg, the size of a golf ball, right at the injection site. Of course, I voiced my concerns again, but the pediatrician insisted this was a mild reaction and quite common, so I pushed my uneasiness down again. If the pediatrician wasn't worried, why should I be worried? Besides, he was meeting his developmental milestones, although at a slower pace. Again, I was assured he was a little slower due to his gender. Boys just develop at a slower pace, I was told, that was all.

When Michael was nine months old, we were referred to an endocrine clinic for some growth and weight issues. The doctor told me that although my son was on the smaller side, he was still growing and gaining weight. My husband and I were both on the shorter side, so it was probably genetic that he was smaller. I questioned his projectile reflux but was again assured that most babies have this and it gets better as they get older. The excuses just kept on coming.

By the time Michael was twelve months old, things took an ugly turn for the worse. I still was uneasy about vaccinating, especially *that* day. He was going to get the MMR. That was the one shot I dreaded. Again, the pediatrician reassured me that the benefit of the shot far outweighed the mild side effects. I really wanted to believe him. My judgment was clouded because Michael was hitting his milestones. He was babbling, saying mama and dada, looked at me, and responded to his name. He didn't have any of the red flags for autism. I was relieved that he was out of the woods, or so I thought. I decided to go ahead with the shots that day, the day after his first birthday. He was vaccinated against MMR, varicella, and hepatitis B all at the same time. He went from a babbling, happy twelve-month-old baby to a thirteen-month-old baby who stopped babbling, stopped saying mama and dada, lost all eye contact, and stopped smiling. He wouldn't respond to his name at all. It didn't sink in right away that something was really wrong, because I just didn't want to admit it to myself. Huge denial. I tried to rationalize that because he was a boy, his skills were a little slower to develop, or he didn't feel well that day, or he was just a quiet kid. My husband questioned whether or not he could hear. The pediatrician said all was fine and there was no hearing loss. I just kept telling myself he was fine. I couldn't bring myself to think that we were going down that dark hole and losing him to autism. The worst part of all was that, ultimately, I was responsible for allowing him to get the shots in the first place. I know people will say it wasn't my fault, that I couldn't have known, and that I was right to listen to the doctors, but it doesn't make the guilt go away. It takes over your soul.

They say autism can shake a marriage to its core, and the next four years for us were a nightmare to say the least. I don't think many couples could have lived through what we had to and keep their marriage intact. Unfortunately, it wasn't just autism we would deal with but also many medical problems and medical procedures before we even got the official diagnosis of autism at three years old. There were things that we couldn't have prepared for as parents or even imagined we would need to learn.

Michael was a late walker. We got the whole speech from the pediatrician that boys do things late and moms tend to do everything for their sons, so they might hit their milestones later. I decided to believe this at first, but mom intuition kept nagging at me. By fifteen months old, Michael still wasn't walking but could cruise furniture really easily. We insisted to our pediatrician that something was not right, and he referred us to a pediatric orthopedist. I knew Michael was having language delays at this point, but I decided to wallow some more in denial and focus on this new curveball of a possible orthopedic problem. This was the first of many, many hurdles we would be forced to face.

"Your son's hips are dislocated." What? How do a child's hips become dislocated? It was a condition called bilateral hip dysplasia, the doctor explained in a very matter-of-fact kind of way. My head was literally swimming at the appointment, and I had trouble focusing on the words that the doctor was telling me. I heard things like "dislocation," "x-rays," "traction," "surgery," "spica cast for six months," "harness." It seemed like a horrible nightmare. The doctor explained to my husband and me that our son would need to be in traction for two weeks and then have a closed reduction of hips, which basically meant that they would have to reinsert his femoral head into his acetabulum, or hip socket. It would be a little bit trickier because he was already fifteen months old and the hip sockets were shallow. He also said something very interesting to me: "Your son has low muscle tone. Has anyone ever told you that before?" Nope. His pediatrician never mentioned it once. When I asked the pediatrician about it at a follow-up visit, he said he did note some low tone but didn't feel it was significant enough to mention. Turns out, low muscle tone is very significant. In fact, low muscle tone is a potential consequence of mercury poisoning. His vaccinations contained mercury, and he was right on schedule from two months to twelve months old, but I wouldn't realize that until much later, when I started researching vaccine injury. I didn't have time to stop and think at all. Our next step was to put him in traction. The two weeks of traction were excruciating. I had a fifteen-month-old active toddler who had to lie on his back with his legs extended into the air and pulled down by weights to help stretch his tendons. I could take him out to eat and bathe, but that was it. Fortunately, we were able to apply the apparatus at home on his crib and didn't have to be in the hospital for it. For two weeks, I sat right next to his crib, untwisting him constantly as he was a little acrobat, doing handstands and twisting and turning all over the place. I did cheat a little bit and take him out of it during the night so he could sleep. The whole time, he was a little trooper. I was a wreck on the other hand, but I never let my son see that. I didn't cry or look worried for him, even though I was dying inside. I put on a brave face for my family and pretended I was strong enough to handle this. At this point, lack of sleep and constant worry reared their ugly heads, and I took everything out on my husband. Everything. All my worry, my fears, my exhaustion, everything. It's a credit to him that he didn't walk out on me during that time. He was a child of divorced parents, and it devastated him when he was younger. He always vowed he would be a full-time father to his kids and a full-time husband to me. He's kept that promise to this day. He has stepped up in ways I can't even begin to describe, all the while being positive and focused on our son's recovery.

Taking Michael to the hospital the morning of his surgery was just awful. I had consultations with the doctor and anesthesiologist, who assured me that everything was going to be fine. He would be under anesthesia for two hours. Little did I know that this anesthesia (and the two times he had to be put under for cast changes) would be another toxic assault on his body. The worst night of my life was the night we brought him home with his hip spica cast on. It was heavy. It went from his mid chest to the tips of his toes and put his legs in a frog leg position so his hip bones would stay in the hip sockets. That night he screamed in fear and tried to pull it off. He looked at both my husband and me with this absolute look of horror on his face that he was stuck in there and couldn't get out. The feeling of utter helplessness was overwhelming. It was one of the most awful experiences of my life to see my child in utter panic, and there was nothing I could do but hold him and rock him to sleep. As the days went on, he got used to crawling on the floor, dragging his heavy cast behind him. He really was such a trooper and adapted well to life in this cast. People would always ask me how he went to the bathroom. Well, there was a cutout where he could pee and poop, but keeping that cast pee-free and poop-free was a challenge. I had to buy infant diapers to insert into the hole cut into the cast and then a bigger diaper outside to put around the cast. I had to change it about fifteen times a day because if the cast got wet, it would stink really badly. At our follow-up appointments, the doctor would comment how the cast didn't smell like most tend to do. Even though it sapped all my energy, I made sure that boy was clean and dry at all times. Because he couldn't fit into his crib with his cast on, I put the mattress on the floor next to the couch and slept next to him for six months. He would wake up quite frequently because it was uncomfortable to sleep that way.

The lack of sleep and the stress about his condition put our marriage on hold for six months. It was like we were in a war and knew when it would be over and just had to fight through every day to get there. I was a walking zombie, and my husband was usually working, so no time for romantic dinners or date nights for us; it was just about survival at that point. When our son's last cast finally came off five months later, the doctor told us Michael would be walking within six weeks. It took five months for him to take his first steps because of the low muscle tone. He took his first steps two weeks after his second birthday. It was the most exciting moment of our lives to that point. To see your child take his or her first steps is exhilarating! I was beginning to think he would never be able to walk.

During this whole time, my husband and I were so focused on his orthopedic progress that we didn't really notice his speech delay. We ditched the old pediatrician as soon as we realized that he had dropped the ball in diagnosing the hip dysplasia too late, and we got a new one. At our initial consultation, the new pediatrician was concerned about Michael's reflux issues. He sent us to a feeding clinic, and at that appointment our son was evaluated by chance for developmental delays. I say "by chance" because the woman who was there that day normally didn't work in that office but was there for another reason. She noticed Michael in the waiting room, introduced herself, and asked if we had any concerns about his development. Still being a little in denial, I said that he was a little slow to hit his milestones, possibly from all his orthopedic issues, and that was holding him back. She did some testing that day, and he qualified for Early Intervention services. I was a little taken aback to be honest. We had just lived through this whole traumatic ordeal and were so happy to have our son out of that cast, and now they were telling me he needs services? Barely able to take a breath from our first hurdle, the next hurdle was upon us.

We started Early Intervention and had the therapists come to our house. I was always optimistic that Michael would be able to catch up and he would grow out of it. Even our family felt that way. It was just the trauma of the surgery that was holding him back. We did home PT, OT, and speech therapy for a year and a half with some modest gains. He was still nonverbal but learned some signs and was able to communicate a little bit. Still no pointing, poor eye contact, and no social skills. I even researched autism on the Internet and knew he had a lot of the red flags, but I still wanted to live in denial and didn't want to believe it was autism. I thought he would just break out of it and join us in our world.

During this time, I became pregnant with my daughter. She was very much unplanned but has been such a huge blessing in our lives and her brother's life. She is very advanced and very social and is determined to pull him out of his isolation every chance she gets. Some days, I wish I had half her energy and determination. Seeing how rapidly she was developing and hitting her milestones made it obvious how far behind Michael was. Even after eighteen months of therapies, we got the dreaded diagnosis the month before his third birthday.

"Your son has autism." I'm not an overly emotional person, but that day those words cut into my very soul. It felt as if there was no air in the room. I burst out in tears; my husband will say more like sobs. I couldn't hold it in. The hopes and dreams we had for our son just vanished with those four words. The psychologist was saying something to me, but I couldn't look at him. What happened to our perfect dream? We were in love, I had found my Prince Charming, and it wasn't supposed to be this way. You ride into the sunset, and you live happily ever after. We had just lived through an absolutely horrible, gut-wrenching experience with the hip surgery, and now I had to hear that my son had autism? I couldn't let myself think what might be next. I couldn't bear to look into my husband's eyes and see the sadness overtake him. Yet again, we had to put on our game faces. I don't think our families knew what to say to us or how to handle the news. Maybe it was too uncomfortable or sad, but for whatever reason, they checked out of our lives for a time. Not to say we didn't talk to them or visit, but the visits were few and far between, and the conversations were centered on their lives and their problems, not on autism.

I was barely functioning, taking care of a colicky baby and a toddler with extreme night terrors, with a husband working second shift. I admit I started to resent him for not being there more. It did start to put a strain on our marriage, but divorce was not something we ever considered. It was a really rough patch. We still loved each other very much, but that idea of the white picket fence and the great life in suburbia was getting further and further out of our reach. It was an enormous struggle, but we had to depend on each other to get through it. I foolishly thought our families would do more to help us out or offer more support, but it didn't happen. Our family felt Michael had autism and that there was nothing we could do. We felt differently. We knew the potential he had and were determined to fight tooth and nail to access it.

Our home ABA program started the month Michael turned three. It was hands down the best therapy for him. The two thera-pists we worked with were just the best teachers and really special people. They truly cared about Michael and even let our daughter participate in his sessions. He really loved them, and we were so sad when the program ended. When our son turned four, we enrolled him in an autism pre-K program that was a forty-five-minute drive away. I would pack up both kids, drive the forty-five minutes, and drop him off. I thought the first day that I was going to throw up. He had never been away from me before; this was our first step into letting our son into the "real world." It was so hard to let his little hand go and trust that the teachers were going to take care of him the way I had all these years. He ended up doing very well in the program. We were so lucky to have come across such caring therapists and teachers in those early years. It made the whole process seem less scary.

That school year ended, and we were faced with the big leap into kindergarten. Pre-K had been a half-day program, and the thought of sending him to kindergarten really made me nervous. He was still nonverbal, and it was completely nerve-wracking to think he would be away from me for a full eight-hour school day. The first day came, and I had to put Michael on the bus. I thought I would go out of my mind that day. I wished I could be a fly on the wall and just watch him to make sure he was okay. The staff and his aide were so good to him, and he was adapting very well into the school setting. It seemed like we were facing these hurdles and knocking them over and finally winning. It started to feel like the fairy-tale dream was still a possibility for us. Our son was doing well, and we started to get excited about the future. And then the other shoe dropped.

"Your son has diabetes." It had to be a cruel joke. It just had to be. My husband is a type 1 diabetic, and one of our fears was that one of our children would develop it. I knew weeks prior that something was not right. Michael was constantly thirsty and urinating all the time and losing weight. We took his blood sugar reading with my husband's glucometer, and it read 549. Normal blood sugar is 80–100. My husband and I just looked at each other and literally made excuses as to why the reading was so high. His hands were sweaty, he was upset and crying, he ate too much fruit that day, etc. We didn't want to face it at all. I didn't sleep that night, knowing that the next day our lives were going to change forever. Again. We took him to the pediatrician's office the next day, and the tests confirmed what we feared. It was diabetes. The doctor instructed us to take him to the local Children's Hospital as soon as possible. I remember getting in the van, buckling the kids up, getting behind the wheel, and just sobbing. It was the first and only time I've ever cried in front of my kids. My daughter asked me why I was crying. She was two at the time but knew something was wrong. Not wanting to worry her, I sucked it up, and we went back home to pack a bag for the hospital and started to make phone calls to our family about what was going on.

My husband is very strong and emotionally tough, especially in emergency situations. He always has a very clear head. He's my "go-to guy" in any sort of panic. I overheard him start to tell his father over the phone, and he couldn't get the words out. He just started to cry. He believed in his heart that he gave him this disease because he had it too, and he blamed himself. We were both utterly devastated. After getting home from the hospital, I had to now test Michael's blood four to five times a day and give him shots four times a day. There were times I wanted to give up. My husband was at work, and I had to wrestle Michael down while he was screaming in fear of this needle, and I had to stick him with it without hurting him or me. The whole experience was a complete nightmare.

Our families didn't understand why we were so stressed. They would be sympathetic from afar, but that was it. I didn't have time to explain the enormity of raising a child with special needs and medical problems, IEP meetings, juggling therapies at school and at home, and having special diets. I didn't have time to say how utterly devastating it was to never hear your child say, "I love you, Mom," or to not know what he is feeling every day. It rips at a mother's heart. I couldn't explain how devastating it was to my husband that he wouldn't see his son play football. Of course, I sucked it all up and just let go of all my frustrations on my husband, who felt helpless himself being away from us at work. I don't think our families realized the enormous amount of pressure that was being put on our marriage. I guess some people choose to run from adversity, and some face it head on. My husband and I faced it head on.

Fortunately, we were blessed with a wonderful daughter. She has been such an incredible sibling to her brother, and her maturity beyond her years has made her able to handle the enormity of her brother's medical conditions. I joke that she could probably run the house and take care of Michael if she ever had to: She's that responsible. Over the years, I've had to rely on her so much, and I thank God every day that she has such a giving spirit and a strong heart like her dad. Autism is hard on parents, but it's also very hard on the siblings. We have had to focus a lot of time and energy on Michael, and Brooklyn sometimes doesn't get as much. When she was little, she didn't understand why her brother didn't talk or why he didn't play with her or look at her. In a lot of ways, she's like an only child. She's had to make some sacrifices throughout the years, but she's never resented her brother for it.

After all this, you would think that we were done with hurdles. Michael had to deal with hip dysplasia, autism, and type 1 diabetes, but there was another hurdle just waiting for us—seizures. Nothing, and I mean nothing, can prepare you for watching your child having a convulsion. It will bring you to your knees. The first seizure happened one July morning. This time, I didn't need a doctor to deliver the bad news; it was right smack in front of my face. My daughter came to wake me up and said her brother was making "monkey noises." I ran into his bedroom and found him convulsing in his bed. My husband was still home; luckily, he had not yet left for work. I carried Michael into the bathroom screaming something was wrong. His body felt like a lead weight. His lips were blue, and his eyes were deviated to the side. He had foam coming out of his mouth. My husband grabbed him, and I ran downstairs in a mad dash thinking he was having a hypoglycemic reaction. I pretty much ransacked my cabinets looking for the glucometer and the glucagon in case I had to administer an emergency shot. The blood sugar was normal, not low. At that point I called 911. It felt like two years before they got to my house. By the time they arrived, Michael had started coming out of it and was crying. The paramedics got him in the ambulance, and I threw on clothes to go with them to the hospital. Just as I was about to run out the door, my daughter stopped me and said, "Mom, I love you." Like I said, this little girl is a gift from God. Amidst all that chaos, she was not the least bit scared. She was there to comfort me and let me know it was all right. God gave Brooklyn to us for that very reason—to let us know God is here with us and giving us his love in the form of a beautiful and wonderful six-year-old girl.

The next two years went by in a blur. There were more 911 calls and more seizures. I took Michael out of school for half a year and decided to homeschool him because the seizures were still not being controlled. He was still able to get his speech and occupational therapy at school. I became a taxicab driver that year. I had to run Michael to speech therapy, drop my daughter at preschool, come back to pick up Michael, go home and do two hours of homeschooling, and then run back out to pick up my daughter. That year was one of the most exhausting of my life. My husband and I barely had time for each other again—no date nights, no dinners, no movies, no vacations. Our date nights became renting a movie on TV and watching half of it before we both passed out. It was difficult listening to stories of our family having fun, excitedly talking about this or that, just picking up and going wherever. We would get the "Hey you're doing a great job" or "God gives special children to special people" lines all the time. Really? Because I think God gives us family who are supposed to be there when times are hard and the chips are down.

I admit it: I became bitter inside, and my relationship with my husband was very up and down; most of the time it was down. When you're fighting for your child, it's really hard to have room for anything else. We both felt neglected and unappreciated. Unfortunately, it was just the nature of the beast. With both of us giving a thousand percent, we were mentally and physically exhausted. Holidays would come and go. My divorced sisters were dating and going out on romantic dinners and overnight getaways, and even getting roses on Valentine's Day. My Valentine's Day gift came from FedEx in the form of a big box of supplements for my son. Flowers and dinners were a luxury we couldn't afford. DAN doctor visits cost us thousands of dollars. Tomatis therapy was $5,000 dollars alone. We had racked up $60,000 in debt, and it bankrupted us. Fortunately, my father-in-law was able to help us out, but it wasn't enough. I wasn't able to really contribute financially, because I had to take care of Michael. It was impossible to just leave him with a sitter or take him to an after-school program, because his needs were too great. Despite all this stress in our lives, we knew that being married and having a loving home was the best thing for our kids. Michael needed both of us, and we couldn't bail on him.

I was pretty depressed at this point that the things we had tried biomedically didn't seem to be helping. I became the Google queen. I did so much research and tried just about everything, but Michael was a tough nut to crack. He was eight years old now, still nonverbal for the most part, and still clearly autistic. The seizures seemed to be causing a regression, which was weighing on me pretty heavily. Right about this time, I started having serious conversations with God. It was a make-or-break time, and I was giving him an ultimatum. Yep, I gave God an ultimatum. I was sick and tired of being a prisoner to autism, diabetes, and seizures. If Michael was going to have any sort of a chance at a life, I needed to get my crap together and find out how to give it to him. That's when we started homeopathy.

I had always wanted to stay more on the natural side of things, and homeopathy seemed to be a good fit for us. I had used it over the years for acute things with good success, and there was a homeopath whom other moms in the autism community were recommending who was having pretty good results. I did the initial consultation via Skype, and it was an experience I will never forget. Very intense. I had to recount my pregnancy and birth experience and things about my son that were very emotional for me. My husband was not on board with this at all, but being the supportive man that he is, he allowed me to pursue it. I thought the man would walk around with a tinfoil hat on if he thought it would help our son. There are some wonderful warrior moms out there, but there are some pretty kick ass warrior dads too, and I happen to be married to one of them.

Homeopathy turned out to be a blessing in more ways than one. God must have been listening to my ultimatum that day because he guided me down a path that has changed my life and my family for the better. Autism can be extremely lonely and isolating for a family. You can't do the things typical kids and families can do. My son couldn't handle most activities. They would just overwhelm his sensory issues. Most days, it was just easier to stay home. When I started homeopathy, I became a member of an online homeopathy support group. I've been part of online groups before, but they were usually run by a few not-so-nice people who enjoyed getting into cyber arguments and petty back-and-forth stuff. This group put aside all negativity and focused on the positive. We all had really crappy stuff going on—challenges with our kids, school, and home—but we found a way to become a really great support system to each other.

God listened to me that day when I asked him to please show me how to help my son and give me the tools to do it. He led me to this group of extremely kind and dedicated warrior moms (and one warrior dad) who opened my eyes to the fact that I was missing out on joy. And laughter. They gave me the strength to get back in the fight and keep going, to leave no stone unturned when it came to Michael's recovery. In the darkest corners of my mind, I believed that it was too late for my son and that he was too old to make any real gains. I started to resign myself to the fact that this was it and we had to accept it and move on. Joining this group was like the sun coming out again. We all had the same mantra: "Autism bites monkey turds!" It does. It bites big-time monkey turds.

For the first time in a long time, I feel hope, and it's had a ripple effect in my life. I had the courage to finally start chelation with tons of help and support. Most importantly, I don't have to dump as much on my husband anymore. I have this wonderful group of people to boost me up from my lowest lows and celebrate my highest highs. Most people use Facebook to brag about themselves or post inane pointless drivel, but Facebook has given me a truly special gift. Who knew God was such a Mark Zuckerberg fan?

Most of all, I realized that autism, diabetes, and seizures aren't the end of the story. With the love, support, and inspiration from my wonderful husband and daughter, I realize every day that there are volumes of empty pages just waiting to be written in Michael's life. My husband and I have faced some pretty big hurdles together, but we've overcome some little ones too. Potty training. Handwriting. Math. Learning letter sounds over and over again until a few words started to emerge. Playing catch. Taking shoes off. Putting clothes on. Brushing teeth. Going to a restaurant without a meltdown. All these accomplishments make my husband and me stronger in our marriage and dedication to each other. With each new milestone comes new resolve. We are more united and more in love today than ever before. We have an unwavering respect for each other and an unwavering love for our children. We may not have the white picket fence or the dog, and I may not be a soccer mom, but what we have is pretty special. I know in my heart that one day I'll get to hear my son say, "I love you, Mom. Thanks for not giving up on me."

THE PROFESSOR'S FRACTURED FAIRY TALE

Once upon a time, I had a fairy-tale family: a king and queen who were crazy about each other, a beautiful little three-year-old princess, and a gorgeous newborn prince. If we could freeze the frame right there, life would always be perfect. Only life isn't like that. (Cue needle scratching a record.) The prince stopped breathing after about thirty-six hours and was put on life support and IV antibiotics to no avail. Before he could make it through forty-eight hours, he was gone. When my daughter cried inconsolably in the NICU, the doctor in charge told her, "Don't worry. Your parents will get you another one." Fortunately, I was in the other room holding my son at the time or my little Zaney might not have been the only one who didn't survive the day.

As a family, we had a very tough time dealing with Zane's death. Losing a child is one of the most difficult things that can happen to anyone, no matter how young the child. It's also one of the most stressful things that can happen to a marriage. Ours was no exception. Everyone grieved differently. Our daughter was spirited, high-strung, and very confused whereas we were depressed and angry. Not a good combination.

In the film *Lilo and Stitch*, Lilo says to her older sister Nani, "We're a broken family, aren't we?" Oh, did that line resonate in our house! My daughter began seeing a therapist (at the whopping age of four) to help her with her over-the-top anxiety. My husband started seeing a therapist, too, because he had gotten so depressed he was having suicidal thoughts. Me? I was just trying to hang on until we could put the pieces of life back together.

I was forty-one when Zane was born, and had always wanted two children. Zane's birth was supposed to be the end of trying to conceive, pregnancy, and childbirth. Bill even planned to get a vasectomy a few weeks later. I felt cheated, almost as if the universe was laughing at me, "You said, 'two children!' You didn't say you had to keep them! Gotcha!"

After many a painful conversation on the subject, my husband and I decided we would try again. But who knew if I had another full-term baby in me? Certainly the clock was ticking and ticking fast. I read the book *Taking Charge of Your Fertility (TCOYF)*, by Toni Wechsler, and joined an online message board community called Ovusoft. It was originally started to help people work with the concepts in the book and the software that was based on it. What I found there was so much more than support for TCOYF. It was really a forum for a vast assortment of women from all over the world to get together and exchange ideas.

At Ovusoft, I encountered a good friend that I'd lost track of after Zane's death (like, oh, say, 85 percent of my life). She belonged to a group of women who were dealing with infertility and all the subsequent treatments that usually implies. Despite the fact that I was not yet dealing with "infertility," she invited me to join her group, and I became a member of Still Standing. In addition, I found another budding group for women who were trying to conceive after a loss. We called it Aching Arms, Hopeful Hearts (AAHH) because we'd all discovered that your arms really *do* ache to hold a baby after you've given birth. (I can't tell you the number of times it was all I could do not to snatch a baby from a passing stroller and run.) The women on those two boards became some of my best friends and, what's more, became my lifelines when things got tough.

Just over two years after Zane died, a friend from Still Standing had a daughter who was stillborn. Lisa was a beloved figure at

Ovusoft, and everyone was eagerly awaiting her daughter's birth. I particularly liked her because she and I were the bleeding-heart liberals on the board. When I heard about her daughter Scarlett, it triggered all the feelings around Zane's death all over again, and I realized that even though I was the "newbie," I was going to be the best help for Lisa as she went through the same nightmare I had experienced. Life has a wicked sense of humor, or irony at any rate, and I actually got pregnant the night Scarlett died, even though technically we were "taking a break" from "trying." I was ten weeks pregnant when I went to visit Lisa in Los Angeles. We had one lovely afternoon and evening, and the next day I miscarried. See what I mean about irony? There was a tremendous amount of blood, a missed flight, and a lot of anguish for poor Lisa who had to take me to the same hospital where she'd said both "hello" and "good-bye" to her beloved baby girl.

That whole experience nearly put me under. I had read somewhere that there were very few spontaneous pregnancies in women over 43, and I was very afraid that miscarriage was the end of the line for me fertility-wise. I started seeing a therapist to help me deal with this new wave of grief and the possibility I wasn't ever going to get another chance.

I was getting older and older and not getting pregnant and not doing much else with my life either. Finally, we decided that since our health insurance would cover one round of in vitro fertilization (IVF) we would try it, and if it didn't work, that would be it; no more trying. On to the next phase of life! I ended up doing the IVF in the last months that I qualified for both the clinic and my insurance. The first attempt was a disaster. They followed a "Lupron flare" protocol and didn't suppress my own cycle enough. I ovulated early, and they canceled the retrieval the night before *without telling me*! I had to call and badger the clinic to find out if I was confirmed. Obviously, that left a more-than-bitter taste in our mouths. But my reproductive endocrinologist (RE) was extremely apologetic. She said that if I wanted, we could do another round of drugs the next month—even though she *never* does back-to-back cycles—because it was the only month I had left to qualify. It was then or never. She promised that there was no way the clinic would mess up again, and she agreed to an Antagon protocol that I thought made more sense for me. I couldn't bear the idea of giving up without doing whatever we could, so we held our noses and dived in again.

The RE was not exactly encouraging. "Rates of success at your age are very low." "Your ovaries are not responding to the drugs." "We'll schedule the egg retrieval, but don't get your hopes up." "You have eight eggs, but they won't all be mature." I tuned out as much as I could and thought to myself, *All it takes is one good one.*

We showed up for the egg retrieval hardly daring to breathe, feeling certain that someone somewhere would yank the rug out from under us. When I woke up in recovery, the nurse told me they'd retrieved nine eggs. I made her repeat it. I thought she'd mixed me up with someone else! When I called the next day for a fertilization report, I was told seven of the nine had fertilized. That was *much* better than I'd been hoping for! I showed up for the three-day transfer, and the doctor told me I still had six embryos and *all* of them had at least eight cells. He said they were good quality, and he wanted to transfer all six because the chances of multiples in my age range were very, very low. We really didn't want twins, but we really did want this to work. So we once again held our noses and let him transfer all six. It was starting to look like we might get another child after all!

Less than two weeks later, I tested positive on a home pregnancy test, and soon after ultrasound confirmed one embryo. Whew! After an anxiety-wracked nine months (including one horrendous late-night trip to the ER when I thought I was leaking amniotic fluid), I gave birth at home to another prince, Bryce. The only drug I had was an IV antibiotic because I tested positive for the group B strep bacteria. I was glad to have it, because Zane had died of a freak strep A infection. Bryce came into the world at 23 in. and 9 lb. even. He was much scrawnier than his brother, who was a whopping 10 lb. 10 oz., at 23 in. Actually, Bryce was different in many ways: His birth was much faster; he had much less vernix, even though he was only two days late; he had much less hair; and he was also the only one of my children who actually cried when he was born. His face was all scrunched up, and he looked like a crotchety old man, but my prince was absolutely beautiful to me.

Bryce grew well and seemed better able to sleep than his older sister, which was a relief. But nursing didn't seem any easier the second time around. It involved a lot of pain (yes, I was doing it right; after the initial horrific three months with my daughter, I nursed her for three years), and there were times I came close to giving up. Just when the pain finally abated, Bryce started having trouble sleeping. His nose would get congested and he would wake up. The congestion seemed to come and go in the beginning, but after a while, it happened more often than not. His pediatrician seemed unconcerned. "I'm sure it's not the breathing. He would just breathe through his mouth." *Well, he's not! He's waking up! Every frigging hour!* At the same time, she berated me for still nursing at night. She was of the firm opinion that three-month-olds should be left to cry it out. (Insert eye roll here.) Clearly, I was going to have to figure this out on my own.

This might be a good time to tell you something about the kind of person I am. "Information sponge" would not be a bad description. I thrive on learning as much about a subject as possible. I'm a mystery lover who has been a contestant on Jeopardy! When I set out to figure something out, I figure it out. I attended one of the most highly selective colleges in the country on a prestigious scholarship and graduated in three years with a degree in Physics. When I took the GRE (because I was applying to graduate acting programs, a whole other side of my personality we won't go into here . . .), I got 800s on the math and logic sections. Logic comes so naturally to me that I was stunned to find out that it was not so for others. That, plus my science background, means that I can read a scientific study and spot the flaws rather easily.

The waking was better some nights than others. It seemed to be much worse after I ate ice cream and pasta meals. If I ate both of them together, we were guaranteed a night of hell. (Yes, I actually tested this.) *Okay, so let's see what happens when I cut out dairy?* Much better. Not perfect, but much better. Then I cut out wheat. Again, much better. We were getting some peaceful sleep hours. He was even starting to sleep longer periods some nights, three or even four hours. But there were still a lot of unexplained not-so-good nights. I realized that Bryce was reacting to other, environmental things. I tried a humidifier to alleviate some of the issues, but it turned out that the humidifier increased the dust and mold in the air, both of which he seemed to react to. He even started to get an asthmatic-type cough. Of course, when I took Bryce back to the doctor, she didn't detect it. She said, "Asthma doesn't just come and go like that." Of course it does. I've had asthma for thirty-seven years now, and I guarantee that for the first few years at least you wouldn't have known it most of the time. I'm allergic to a lot of things, and when I'm not being exposed to them, I'm fine. She seemed to think he couldn't be allergic to dust because he'd be sick *all* the time and not just in bed at night. Well, I'm allergic to dust, and I'm not sick all the time!

Once Bryce had a bad ear infection. Naturally enough, given our history, I panicked when my normally easygoing son went off the deep end. It was evening, so I took him to the hospital, and they gave him antibiotics that seemed to make him better. I was grateful.

Another, seemingly minor thing was that even though Bryce started eating solid food at six months, and a lot of it, he never had formed stools. I was used to gushy stools from breastfeeding, so it was a few months before I realized how odd that was. Again, the pediatrician was unconcerned. "I could send him to a gastroenterologist if you like, but do you really want to do invasive testing?" No, I didn't. But surely there was *something* I could do about it?

When Bryce was about fifteen months old, a cousin told me about her daughter's food allergies at a Christmas party. She'd taken her daughter to a chiropractor who did an allergy elimination technique involving acupressure. I was desperate, so I set up an appointment without even researching it, because I knew acupressure couldn't hurt him. The technique was called NAET (Nambrudripad's Allergy Elimination Technique), and nobody can explain why it works in a way that makes sense to a logical mind, but it *does* work. I took both kids, eventually, but the difference in Bryce's sleep after a couple of months of treatments was night and day. Turned out, he was naturally a really good sleeper!

In the meantime, I kept expecting him to start talking. He babbled like the books say. (My daughter, Trinity, didn't, so I thought
this was a great sign.) I remember thinking when Bryce was a few
months old that this guy was going to be an early talker because he
just seemed to want to communicate so badly. At nine months, he
came out with "dada," and we thought we were golden. His sister
hadn't said "mama" till she was twelve months old, and she is, and
was, an incredibly verbal child (though she did have some significant
articulation issues the first few years). Unfortunately, Bryce didn't
really add to his early success. Every once in a while, he would say
something that would take us by surprise. I remember once he said,
"Doggie!" while pointing at a dog, but no matter what we tried, we
couldn't get him to repeat it. Another time, I was playing with him
and he said, "Peek-a-boo!" clear as could be. Again, we couldn't
get him to repeat it. In fact, he was about three before we could get
even "Peek-boo" out of him again.

This was mystifying and frustrating to me (imagine how it felt to
him!). At the age of fourteen months, Bryce seemed to start adding
"words." He had four syllables that he used to refer to some things.
(I misplaced my list of words when we moved. That's probably
good; it usually depresses me to read it.) Then, Bryce got a second
ear infection, and this time he got an antibiotic with a higher dose.
At sixteen months, he had four words—different words than he'd
had at fourteen months! At eighteen months, he *still* wasn't talking,
and I knew there was something wrong. I wanted to get on top of
it as soon as possible so it wouldn't mess up his early school years.
I regretted not getting help for Trinity's articulation until she was
four as she responded so well to speech therapy when she got it.

Bryce had a hearing test, which he passed with flying colors,
though his ears still bore some mark (negative pressure) of his previous ear infection. Then, at nineteen months, we had him evaluated
for the Early Intervention (EI) program here in New York City.
The therapists were sweet, but they let me know that he had to be
at least 33 percent delayed in one area before he could qualify for
services. Expressive speech was definitely delayed by enough, but
that score was going to be lumped in with the receptive language

score to determine an overall score in this "one area." Bryce was not at his best that day, so they could be forgiven for not believing me when I said, "He understands *everything!*" However, even on a bad day, he was never going to score 33 percent behind on receptive language. One of the examiners tossed off a comment that I didn't pick up on right away. She said, "There is a disorder called apraxia that is characterized by normal receptive language but difficulty with expressive language. If I were to diagnose it now, though, I would be laughed out of the profession."

True to their predictions, Bryce did not qualify for EI, but I was encouraged to come back when he was twenty-four months old, because at that point the criteria changed, and expressive delay would be enough to qualify. In the meantime, his language still wasn't progressing. So, I took Bryce to his sister's old speech therapist, and we paid for it out of pocket. This was the best damned speech teacher in the universe, and even *he* wasn't getting anywhere with Bryce. At one point, the therapist told me, "He's very self-aware. I've never known a child this age to be so conscious of his own issues. Bryce won't even try, because he *knows* how hard it is for him." He was twenty-two months old.

Around this time, I had begun randomly, and perhaps a bit desperately, Googling speech issues in young children. I came up with websites dedicated to childhood apraxia of speech. Childhood apraxia of speech is a speech-planning disorder. In other words, the brain knows what it wants to say, but can't figure out how to get the mouth to say it. As soon as I read a description of the disorder, I thought, "Holy shit! That's him!" The prognosis for it wasn't good. They recommended *intense* speech therapy five days a week, with a particular technique called PROMPT, which stands for prompts for restructuring oral muscular phonetic targets. Even given that, they didn't make any claims about how well your kid would talk. As a matter of fact, they implied that speech would *always* be difficult. I admit I panicked a bit.

Fortunately for all concerned, my old friend from Still Standing asked me one day if I had considered apraxia. I couldn't believe she'd even heard of it. "Yes! That's what I think it *is!*" She asked if

I would be interested in being put in touch with some friends who were dealing with apraxia as well. My friend had twin boys born almost exactly one year before Bryce's birth (and actually born on Zane's birthday). One of the boys had been diagnosed with PDD-NOS the year before, and she had subsequently joined an Ovusoft group for moms of kids with autism. Some of these women were dealing with dual diagnoses of autism and apraxia.

It turned out that both mothers were women I had encountered in other boards. One was a member of AAHH, and the other was on a board for liberals who wanted a safe place to discuss politics. One woman mentioned omega-3s and told me she was still nursing and took a lot of cod liver oil to give her son the omega-3s he needed. Well, I was still nursing, too, and I had fish oils on the shelf. I immediately upped my intake, and suddenly many more words were popping out. Even better, Bryce finally started building on what he could do. I was already greatly encouraged.

When the other woman told me that she was "healing her son's gut" because of antibiotic damage, I said, "Whoa! I need some explanation on this." I had suspected that Bryce's repeated exposure to antibiotics messed with his ability to speak, and we knew he had digestion issues! She directed me to some people who explained the gut-brain connection, and they gave me a number of suggestions on how to begin, as well as several book recommendations, including *Enzymes for Autism and Other Neurological Conditions*, by Karen L. DeFelice; *Gut and Psychology Syndrome*, by Natasha Campbell-McBride; *Healing the New Childhood Epidemics*, by Kenneth Bock, MD; and *The Late Talker*, by Marilyn C. Agin and Lisa F. Geng. I read them all and started Bryce on digestive enzymes when he was just over two. As soon as we began, even though we started "low and slow" as recommended, we saw *immediate* gains. Bryce's first real sentence came a few days into this process.

An unexpected byproduct of this exploration and education was that I recognized my daughter in the pages of several of the books. I had wondered about her and the possibility of ADHD before, but all the descriptions I had read previously implied that she didn't really qualify. These books had slightly different criteria and made it clear she *did* qualify. Not only that, there were things I could do biomedically to help Trinity as well.

Midway through Kenneth Bock's book, I was shocked to find an eerily accurate description of Trinity's behavior in his ADHD chapter. In that section, he discussed a syndrome named PANDAS (pediatric autoimmune neuropsychiatric disorders associated with streptococcal infections). It's a neurological condition triggered by strep infections. The mechanism is similar to rheumatic fever, but instead of attacking the heart, the antibodies attack the ganglia at the base of the brain, resulting in some characteristic obsessive and/ or compulsive behaviors. This explained why Trinity's behavior worsened so dramatically at times. Messages would be blocked by the inflamed ganglia and become like a broken record (I know that analogy is lost on the youngsters) where the needle can't move on and it goes in the same groove over and over and over again. I immediately started her on enzymes, fish oils, and some supplements aimed at calming her anxiety and obsessive thoughts. There was overnight improvement with her as well.

The other unexpected byproduct of my education process was that I discovered that Bryce's health history was shockingly similar to that of many of the children with autism I knew. He had food allergies, ear infections, and antibiotics in his background. It seemed that every day I was hearing of another child who'd had the same progression, but almost all of them were more severely affected. Why?

When Trinity was a toddler, I started hearing rumbling about possible problems with the MMR vaccine. So, I held off on that shot while I investigated the rumors. That led to an investigation of vaccines in general. The more I learned, the sorrier I was that I'd ever had her vaccinated at all. For instance (just the tip of the iceberg) the hepatitis B vaccine is for a blood-borne illness transmitted by the same pathways as AIDS—sexual activity or sharing dirty needles. And yet three doses of this vaccine are "required" for all infants at birth, one month, and six months. How many babies do you know who are having sex or sharing dirty needles? Me? I don't know any. And the vaccine-induced immunity wears off before any of those children *are* having sex or sharing dirty needles. So we have spent a fortune vaccinating an entire generation for something they are extremely unlikely to be exposed to, only to have the "protection" wear off before it might do any good. That's fine, we can throw our money away as a country if we choose if the vaccine—as doctors vow—does no harm. But is that the case? Well, when my daughter was vaccinated, the shots still contained a whopping dose of mercury. In addition, a recent Stonybrook study analyzed National Health Interview Survey 1997–2002 datasets and found a nearly three-fold incidence of autism spectrum disorders in boys vaccinated for hepatitis B. If that's not enough to make you stop and question everything you ever thought about vaccines, I don't know what is. I've read the studies that supposedly show that vaccines have no connection to autism, and I can tell you that they do nothing of the sort. First, the "conclusion" of the study is usually "inconclusive," which is "proof" of exactly nothing. Second, most studies are so badly designed that you could drive a truck through the holes in them. They appear to be designed in order to get a non-statistically significant result so that the researchers can say they are "inconclusive." As a result, Bryce has had no vaccines at all. Given the comparison between his health history and that of my friends' children, I'm convinced that the only thing standing between him and autism was his mother's refusal to vaccinate.

I took Bryce back to get evaluated again. This time it took longer to coordinate things as his second birthday took place right when everyone was away on vacation, so I couldn't set up appointments. This was worrisome because Bryce was improving so much on the supplements, I thought he might not qualify again. But I knew he needed the therapy.

Bryce finally qualified for EI at about twenty-seven months of age and started three days per week with a new therapist who had been trained in PROMPT, though I never saw her use it. He was still seeing his old therapist twice a week, for which we continued to pay out of pocket. He was getting speech therapy for a total of five forty-five-minute sessions per week. While I had watched Trinity progress rapidly with her speech therapy, that was not the case with Bryce. All of his big gains followed new biomedical interventions. They did not seem in any way correlated to the intensive speech therapy he was receiving. There were even times when his therapists couldn't get him to speak at all, and they would look to me to get him going. It made me realize how vitally important it was for Bryce to continue on our biomedical path. I was convinced that he wanted *very* much to talk with us and was mortified at how difficult it was for him. Every day, he ran into children who could talk a blue streak without any effort at all.

Ovusoft, my lifeline for like-minded women, closed down briefly (and suddenly) in order to change a number of policies. Many people jumped ship during that time period, and I was a little afraid that I might lose the support I had for this journey. (It sure didn't help that this occurred about the same time that my soon-to-be ex-husband began his many business trips to Stockholm, which was pretty much the beginning of the end for the royal couple. What kind of fairy tale was this?) However, I noticed that there was a mass migration to Facebook within the next few months. I'm an old fogey, but what the hell? I joined, too. It took me a while to get up to speed, but it soon had its own rhythm and momentum. I never sought out parents of kids with autism, but I found myself being "friended" by more and more autism moms (and sometimes dads) whenever I commented on vaccines or apraxia.

I have a long history of using homeopathy for intractable health issues. I even have a pretty good stash of remedies at home for colds, nosebleeds, motion sickness, and other acute situations. I was pretty sure homeopathy could be helpful for both my kids, and I had briefly taken them to a homeopath when Bryce was a baby and dealing with the food allergies. The improvement was hit or miss (more miss with Bryce), the process slow, and he had me coming back with both of them every five weeks. It was getting expensive to get no results. In my searches, I had run across a homeopath who specialized in autism and considered getting in touch with him, but his initial consultation was pricey. Plus, I didn't know if he treated other kinds of issues.

I mentioned the homeopath to my friend with the twins, and she decided to try him. She and a couple of others I had gotten to know through Facebook went to see him, and all of their children improved rather dramatically. These were children who had had a lot of biomedical interventions already, but the homeopathy seemed to be just what they needed to complete the recovery process. Others started noting their success, too, and suddenly there was a long waiting list for appointments. I was told that autism wasn't a necessary condition to become a patient, so I made my daughter an appointment about three months down the road. After the appointment, I was invited to join a Facebook group for people using homeopathy to recover their children from autism. I was suddenly interacting on a daily basis with a whole new group of autism parents. It was a very lively group with a lot of traffic. Personally, I loved being able to talk about homeopathy with people who were excited about using it. (That's when Tex came up with "Professor" for my nickname. Remember the "information sponge"?) Much as people liked the opportunity to bounce ideas off each other in quick succession, the group soon got too big for its britches and migrated to another site. I personally don't do well with that type of group. The security tends to mess me over, making me take extra steps just to get where I want to go, and then the setup just isn't user-friendly. I missed Facebook. Turned out, I wasn't the only one, as I was soon invited to another Facebook group, which wasn't a strictly homeopathy-related group, but most of the members met because of homeopathy.

Homeopathy has been alternately wonderful and frustrating for my daughter, but so far it has been terrific for Bryce. His speech was already greatly improved by the treatments we'd done and his strong desire to communicate, but when we started seeing a homeopath at four and a half, he still had a number of missing consonant sounds. Quite soon after we began, speech became startlingly clear to the point that a number of people commented on it. Being understood by the general public boosted Bryce's confidence when talking to others, especially people he didn't know. I've been struck a number of times in recent weeks at the difference in him in social situations. We had a play date at our house recently with four children (including Lisa's twins) he'd never met before, all around his age and all playing with his toys. Bryce was a wonderful host, demonstrating toys and explaining how they worked and making announcements when necessary. My original instincts were right on target, as he loves to talk. At five now, he's a great storyteller with a wicked command of idiomatic expressions and is astoundingly good at putting difficult concepts into words. He still has a little trouble with the "s" and "sh" sounds, is pale as can be, and has some lingering digestive issues, but we've come so far that I know we can go the rest of the way.

Sometimes I wonder about how I came to be so deeply involved with autism parents, given that I don't have any children "on the spectrum." Personally, I have come to believe that "the spectrum" is really much broader than we think it is. Yes, maybe my children are not classified with autism (and I hope they never will be!), but both have (or had) neurological impairments that are helped by similar treatments and, in all likelihood, caused by similar processes. In fact, I now believe that most, if not all, of the modern chronic illnesses so prevalent today have similar roots. As autism numbers have risen, so have those for diabetes, asthma, ADHD, arthritis, life-threatening allergies, obesity, and a number of other autoimmune illnesses. Children with autism really are the "canaries" that are letting us know that so much of our lives has become poisonous to humans, particularly developing humans.

When I was growing up, I didn't know anyone with autism. Seriously. Not anyone. I read every book I could get my hands on about autism. It wasn't hard; there weren't many. Every parent reported doctors who were stumped. They'd never seen the particular set of symptoms before. Diagnosis took a while because the doctors had no idea what it was. Now, it seems that every other person I know, even those I knew before I got involved with "autism parents," has a child on the spectrum. Given that circumstance, it shocks me to see how many people have their heads buried in the sand. Frequently, I see articles saying that the rise in autism rates isn't real, that autism occurs in the same kind of numbers now that it always has; it's just being *diagnosed* more. Well, that's just not true. I remember the '60s very clearly, and nobody was worried about whether or not his or her children were ever going to potty-train, or speak, or function in a mainstream classroom (and that was back when we had thirty kids sitting in rows), or be able to make a living as an adult, much less all of the above, unless those children had been deprived of oxygen or were born with an extra chromosome. Readers, do your own research! It doesn't take a lot of networking to start seeing underlying patterns in the kinds of health issues plaguing us these days.

I recently met up with a Facebook friend whom I hadn't seen since college. We've discovered with our various posts that we really should have gotten to know each other much better back then, so we're making up for lost time. One of the things we've noticed is a similarity in thinking on health-related topics. She asked about the evolution of my thinking, and as I told her about Ovusoft and the various networks of women I'd met there, she exclaimed, "You're an early adopter! You've been social networking for years!" I'd never thought of it that way, but I guess it's true. I am eternally grateful to the universe for guiding me to all the wonderful people who have helped me on this journey, with special mention to the Thinking Moms (and Dad!) writing this book with me who have been such a blessing in my life and that of my children right from the very beginning. I am honored and humbled to have a place among them, and I pledge to do what I can to pay their love and generosity forward. With magical people like this on my side, I can't imagine how my fairy tale can end with anything but "happily ever after."

Bytes from the Count

I went to see a special-needs soccer game for the first time. A kid kicks the ball. The coaches tell two other kids to run after the ball. The kids run up to the ball. The first kid doesn't stop, he keeps running—past the ball . . . off the field, and just keeps going, Forrest Gump style. The adults run after him. The other kid stops at the ball, picks it up, and starts licking it. I look the other way, and the goalie has wandered off the field. He's hugging a tree. Holy shit. I didn't know whether to laugh or cry at it all.

DATE NIGHT WITH THE REV

My husband's name is David Michael Peter Goes. I have been calling him by this name both in times of delight and in exasperation since the day he proposed—which also happened to be the day we met. Just under three weeks after September 11, *the September 11*, we were married in a quaint church at a destination wedding in front of twenty-two family members and friends. As of this writing, we have three children: Madeleine, six; Noah, four; and Liam, two. About three years ago, we landed in the familiar Midwest, just down the street from my in-laws. They still live in the house where Dave grew up, just over a mile from our incomplete subdivision.

On a dreary late winter Friday in 2011, we had no intention of having our usual date night. Plans had already been made for us to attend an art opening for one of Dave's friends the next evening. Two nights out in one week just doesn't happen. But this was a particularly difficult week for us both, and we needed some time to connect, just the two of us. On a whim, he decided to text our babysitter before work to see if she was free.

She was.

The day began as most days do. Liam was singing, "Maaah-mee! Maaah-mee!" looking for a boost out of his crib. Noah, our son with autism, slammed his body into his door, attempting to pop off the flimsy plastic tie we use to tether it shut. The sound of it giving way alerts us to his activity. We use it to prevent him from night wandering and escaping the house, something he attempts daily. Madeleine was snoring, her arms and legs outstretched like a drunken pop star. The night before she was up until nine o'clock watching the *Good Night Show* on Sprout, an hour past her regular bedtime. Dave let me know about our dinner plans for the evening (a pleasant surprise) before heading down to the basement to start a fire and get his day of conference calls started. A Friday morning like any other; except, on this particular morning, I woke up five minutes late.

I hurriedly freed the boys and told them I was happy to see them, gushed about how lucky I am to be their mom, and showered them with kisses. Mads received a sloppy smooch after I tousled her bed head and told her she was beautiful. "Better get moving, Beauty, because the day has lots in store for you!" I like to start their mornings this way because the real world and real life will fill up their heads with lies soon enough. The rapid pace of the digital era makes the window of time we have to fill them up with truth and love seem more like a keyhole.

Noah emerged from his closet out of sorts. He was scratching his legs and had a red rash on his left cheek. That meant the yeast was back. Not good. He stumbled and frowned and was not making eye contact, which was unusual for him. Although he is four, he still drinks from a bottle. It's the only way we can guarantee he is actually ingesting all his medicine, which is imperative given the horrific state of his bowels and his mitochondrial and immune system damage. The mainstream medical community likes to call his condition a "dysfunction," but that is an inaccurate term. The proper definition for what happened to Noah is "damage." You don't take your crumpled car into the shop for repairs after an accident and say, "Can you have a look at my car? I sustained some bumper dysfunction after a drunk driver rammed into me." It was fine before; it's crumpled now. It's damaged. Period.

Anyway, the concoction of medicine, biomedicine, rice milk, and reverse osmosis water tastes awful, but if it comes in a bottle, he will drink it. This morning he really wanted it. From his roost at the top of the stairs, I could tell he'd soaked through his diaper and saturated his pajamas. He anxiously shouted, "Bottle!" as he poked at his wet midsection. Oh, Lord. I did not have the bottle prepared. It goes like this, "Good morning, little man (kiss, pat the tush). Did you sleep well? (Make him look at me and encourage some sort of response.) Here's your bottle, bud! Ten minutes until we get dressed! Big day!" That's how we do it. Every day.

But I overslept today. Five minutes. Stupid, stupid woman.

He ran into his sister's room and began tearing things off the shelves. Smashing framed pictures on the ground and chanting, "No, Noah! No throw! Sorry, Noah, sorry!" He tore through the space like the Tasmanian devil. I shooed him out and locked her door behind me, mentally noting where all the glass was and grabbing her uniform for school. She'd have to get dressed downstairs. Noah threw his body into the door and screamed, "Key! Key!"

When he gets to this level this quickly, it is usually short-lived. It's simply a matter of employing damage control for that powerfully charged span of time, removing the other children, making sure he doesn't harm himself, and ensuring his immediate vicinity is safe. I knew if I could just get him the bottle, I could change his diaper while he drank it, and he would calm down. "No, Noah!" he kept repeating as he chucked matchbox cars, his brother's blanket, and puzzle pieces down the steps. He retreated into his room and emerged with a large plastic bat cave, running at top speed toward the banister. Mads was sitting on the couch just below and would have been seriously injured had he been successful. I screamed bloody murder as I wrenched the toy out of his hands just before launch. That was the last straw. He fell to the floor, kicking and screaming in a full-blown fit of rage.

"Mommy, what wrong with Noah?" asked Liam, as he wiped his puffy eyes, his morning toddler hair resembling a spent firecracker. I explained that Noah just wanted a bottle and everything would be fine. We just had to stay out of his way until he'd finished his tantrum. He nodded in agreement and bent over to retrieve the blanket Noah had thrown on the stairs. In what felt like slow motion, I watched as he plummeted, head first, down ten steps. Another horror-film-caliber scream issued by yours truly.

He was shaken and sobbing. I examined him from head to toe over and over, while my heart pounded in my throat. No dilated eyes or faraway looks, just loud consistent cries. What was I doing, again? Time was ticking. What about that sense of urgency I had before this? What was it . . . ? Oh, the damned bottle! I looked at the clock and realized the school bus would be waiting outside my door in approximately eighteen minutes. No one was dressed; Mads was the only one fed. Noah was momentarily silent amidst the hubbub.

I rushed into the kitchen and poured the various ingredients while mentally flogging myself.

What is wrong with me? I have no one to blame. I wasn't even sleeping—I was lying there awake! Why didn't I just get up? Where is the vitamin D? Which probiotic are we on this week? Too much Modifilan. If he can taste it, he'll spit it out. Add more Coromega. Where is the tyrosine? What dose are we up to with the chelator? What did Dave do with the damned biomed schedule? I better not find the nystatin on the pill shelf and the L-carnitine in the refrigerator or heads are going to roll. There is no way I am going to have time to crush the vitamin C, he'll have to go without it this morning.

"Noo-aah?" I called, as I balanced a still-weary Liam on my hip, vigorously shaking the bottle with my free hand. "Nooo-aahh?" We bounced up the stairs, Liam repeating, "Where Noah, Noooah?" Upon arrival, we found him on the catwalk by the master bedroom, completely naked and frantically grasping two wrought iron rails, trying to fling his body over the banister. No fear, just sheer determination, on a mission to descend seventeen feet onto the hardwood floor of our foyer. The warm affection with which I'd awakened the brood disintegrated. I became an army sergeant on a mission to keep my troops alive.

Kids with autism have superhuman strength when they are committed to a particular outcome. You have to understand, and if you are a parent of a child with autism, I think you will: At times like this—they go away. Their eyes do not show you their souls, their minds are not functioning, and their bodies are producing energy at such a ferocious pace and with such intent that you know your role in whatever is coming next is somewhat irrelevant. God is going to have to help them—and you. You don't reason with a child (or an adult for that matter) with autism in a state of meltdown. You make his or her area safe and wait for it to pass. But, at this particular moment, he was unwittingly trying to kill himself. Clearly, I had to engage. I set Liam aside, crouched down, tackled Noah at the waist, and in one swift motion hurled him onto our bed.

He kicked me repeatedly with the gusto of a cage fighter. But more importantly, he was safe. Mission accomplished. My own adrenaline surge prevented me from any dramatic displays of angst. What good would it have done anyway? "Oh!!!! Ouch! Noah, you kicked mommy in the face. We don't do that." Meaningless. In his world, words mean nothing. Someone stood between him and his goal, that someone was me, and I had to be stopped by any and all means necessary. If I could just get him downstairs to the playroom, to the DVD player, this would all be over. I got him dressed and kept him away from the banister, but he persisted with the kicking and grunting like a captive wolverine, all the way down the steps. Frankly, the stairs terrify me, and I've grown to detest them. One wrong kick could send us both tumbling south. We reached the playroom, and thank God, something was finally going right because *Cars*, his favorite movie, was queued up. Like an addict feeling the sweet relief delivered by a long-awaited needle, his body softened. I handed him his bottle. His rage disintegrated, and a huge smile consumed his tear-stained face as he shouted, "McQueen!"

Ka-chow! It was over. The other two joined him on the couch, and they sat side by side with rapt attention—eyes like saucers—watching a movie they've seen hundreds of times, sucking on their sippies and bottle like three little Maggie Simpsons.

It was at precisely this moment that King David decided to make an appearance. "What is going on up here? Did you not remember I had a seven thirty conference call with my client in Italy?"

Dave has many wonderful qualities. Sincerity and integrity top the list. I love him, of course, but I also admire him. All marriages have their rhythms and complexities, and ours is typical in that regard. Faith, laughter, respect, and forgiveness are the cornerstones. However, on this particular morning, his praiseworthy traits and the generally harmonious nature of our marriage were not the focus of my thoughts. He was questioning me, implying I should have done a better job of keeping the kids quiet, without knowing I was doing everything in my power just to keep them alive.

Seriously? Seriously? *You have* no idea . . .

"I have to get them ready for school right now, and we are way behind schedule." My tone implied that maybe he was cheating on me or, perhaps, gambling away our life savings. I was shaking as I orbited the whole lot of them, picking up socks, stray food fragments, and those stupid, stupid toy soldiers.

The contented angels smiled at the site of him and shouted, "Daddddy!" Little shits.

Really, logic has no home in our household. It didn't matter that Dave was down in that basement making a living so we can keep this house, pay for the kids' schooling, and just have a standard of living in general. Because of Noah's many sensitivities, we have to eat organic—real organic, not USDA organic. That kind of organic is like smoking Camels instead of Lucky Strikes. The hard-to-come-by, real, expensive food, coupled with Noah's therapy and medical bills, costs more than the mortgages on both our properties. Yet he never bitches about this. He never complains about any of the sacrifices he's had to make. He flies from coast to coast on private jets with CEOs, entertaining the upper echelons of our country's most prominent financial institutions. He works with people who summer in French Polynesia and spend their hiatuses on cruises that last for weeks on end. We are frequently invited to Napa for the weekend, to visit his colleagues' summer homes, to "fly in" for marathons, events, concerts. These things that exist on the periphery of his professional life have no place within our familial reality. He always declines graciously and somehow vacillates between these two powerfully contrasting worlds with an ease I could never emulate. Our last vacation destination was fabulous downtown Cleveland. Our son's stay at the luxurious Cleveland Clinic included multiple neurological and genetic tests, for which he was anesthetized and restrained. No pool, no room service, and the night nurses were self-absorbed bitches who could not understand we did not want to hear them trashing their co-workers while they munched on Doritos at two o'clock in the morning.

He comes home to a wife that is frequently unshowered, pissed off, and stressed out. The walls of his 5,000 sq. ft. home are covered, quite literally, in shit. Where there isn't shit, new or old, there is crayon or "washable" marker. Our lovely Tommy Bahama knock-off couch acts as a permanent home to endless loads of clean laundry in need of folding. The kitchen is almost always destroyed, toys and food littering the floor, dishes perpetually in the sink and in the dishwasher. The money he makes is spent on therapies and treatments before it even hits our bank account. Even with the help we have, the cycles in our house are too rapid and intense for any one person to keep the pace. The crowning glory of our home, bought at the height of the market, was supposed to be the walkout man-cave basement. Construction on it was scheduled to start last summer, but that never happened. Autism happened. He works in a freezing-cold concrete dungeon that magnifies the sounds of petulant children from above better than any Bose sound system I've ever heard.

No, he never ever complains about any of this. How is that possible? It doesn't matter anyway, the jerk. I was alone with our children as the morning's events unfolded. They could have been seriously hurt, and it would have been my fault. I've never been one to blame, but the experience of caring for small children and the perpetual stress associated with autism have flicked a switch in my psychological make-up that now allows me this neurotic indulgence, guilt free. Yes, by virtue of his absence, he was indeed responsible for this morning's drama. And he knew it. Without a word, he just gave me a hug and a pat on the back that implied he was aware. Something could have happened. It's too much to bear sometimes.

"We'll talk about it tonight," I said, as I glanced at him sideways over a heap of clean warm laundry.

As the day unfolded, I did what moms do. When Liam went down for his nap, I walked the entire house, taking a mental inventory of every potential danger. I obsessed about how the morning could have turned out differently. I awfulized and ruminated. I walked the catwalk over and over and over again, jiggling the rails to determine their stability, trying to figure out how to prevent this sort of thing from happening in the future. That's it. We'll have to drywall the staircase. Get rid of the wrought-iron rails and the wood banisters. That's all there was to it. What next? The door off the kitchen that was supposed to lead to a sunroom is, instead, flanked by 4 ft. x 4 ft. of pressure-treated wood that crowns fourteen stairs held together with rusty nails. The whole debacle, slammed together to meet building codes on a tight deadline, was structurally sound the year we moved in but has been separating from the house inch by inch ever since. Somehow, someway, that dangerous eyesore had to go. But what goes in its place? Do we drywall over the door, too? Realistically, there is no way we are going to be seeing a sunroom in our future. This was getting depressing. All the things we liked about this house had to go. No time for a pity party; I had to keep going. The back and front doors. The extra-hook top locks we have in place are flimsy, and Noah's learned how to stack objects and use the broom handle to jimmy them loose. Not acceptable. The window cranks have to go. Windows cannot be opened, as it is never safe to have an open second- or third-floor window around a child who screams, "Outside! Outside!" on an hourly basis. The gate. The gate that separates us from Noah's paramour, the pond, is too dainty. It looks nice, but it's not going to prevent him from getting out. The lock is poorly constructed, and the slats are already bent from his previous escape attempts. The prospect of itemizing the multitude of things wrong with our basement, and the tragedy known as our garage, proved too daunting. No worries, though. I experienced an epiphany.

We had to move. Yes! That was the solution. The market was tough, but we could do it. We Goeses do all sorts of crazy things when we set our minds to it. Yes, moving to a small, practical ranch on a tiny, easily monitored and fenced-in lot of land was indeed the solution! Done! We'll call our realtor tomorrow. I couldn't wait to tell Dave.

After a long, much-needed shower followed by a thorough and thoughtful make-up application, I put the finishing touches on a hairdo that did not require a rubber band and crammed myself into skinny jeans. I wanted to look as hot as possible when pitching my fabulous new money-saving idea to my husband. I am such a good wife, I thought, *Looking good, coming up with great ideas.* I wasn't even mad at him for earning a living anymore. All was well. Change was on the way.

We arrived at the restaurant, and within minutes I was savoring an outstanding Pinot Gris in an elegant glass. It was so delicate and simple it reminded me that sometimes I miss possessing lovely things. With a big enthusiastic smile, I dropped the bomb. "So, what do you think about downsizing? Maybe . . . moving."

"What—what did you just say?" Dave asked as he took a larger than usual gulp of his double vodka martini with a glossy blue-cheese-stuffed olive. His appreciative smile faded.

"Just hear me out . . ." I talked about the necessary drywall, the stairs, what happened that morning, and so many other mornings when he was traveling and I was on my own. I went on to complain and moan about every single aspect of the house—the home we worked together for years to build. I kvetched about everything from the plumbing to the ventilation, the crappy kitchen sink, and the cracks in the drywall. And the safety hazards . . . Why, we were lucky the damn place hadn't been condemned! Everything was just so hard for me. I couldn't even take the kids outside in the summer, because I couldn't keep track of all of them in that huge yard with three points of entry that we can't afford to landscape or finish. We can't do anything in this beast of a house. Let's cut our losses. Living on the pond, we know what a nightmare that's become. And the view of the park outside our dining room window is pure hell because Noah is always stimming—self-stimulating—off of it, screaming "Park, park!" Blah, blah, blah. It will never do. We needed a ranch. A humble, no-frills ranch. Which we could get for a song. We could sell the Escalade. I don't need anything fancy anymore. Those days are gone. No high-maintenance wife here; no, Sir. Just the necessities, that's how I roll. You may thank me for my brilliance now.

His drink was completely gone by the time I'd completed my monologue. His eyes were squinting, and his fingers interlocked over his lips, obscuring his expression. He released his grip on his mouth and yelled at me like I was a toddler who'd just stolen the remote and switched channels during the last pitch of the World Series.

"Why are you doing this to me? Are you kidding me? Why would you drop this on me right now? You have got to be kidding. How long have you been thinking about this? What in God's name is wrong with you?"

The questions weren't what bothered me. It was the fact that he was scolding me. We had raised our voices at one another approximately four times before this altercation, and I can remember each and every time like it was yesterday. Embarrassed, deflated, and angry, I started to cry.

"Why are you yelling at me?" I stammered out as I tried to get control of the water flowing from my sparkly, lined eyes. "I am not responsible for Noah's autism." Ha! Even I didn't believe that one. I completely hold myself responsible for his autism. Knowing what I know now, it is impossible not to—but that's a good thing because I also hold myself responsible for his recovery.

"No! No, you do not get to turn this around on me! I am not blaming you for autism; I'm blaming you for this suggestion. You think we can just get up and move? What the hell are you thinking? No, you don't get to cry right now. Do *not* do this right now!" He slammed his fist on the table.

Dave is a large, athletic man. He still works out every morning, and his biceps are the size of Popeye's forearms. Normally they are quite dreamy. Right now, and for the first time in our nine-year marriage, I was a little afraid of them. He did not answer my question. He pursed his lips and looked down at the floor. Being the woman I am, I assumed that meant I should fill the silence.

"Control your tone, and get a hold of yourself. What the hell is wrong with you?" I hissed. "Do you think I want this? Do you think I want to just scrap our lives and start over? We don't have a choice. He's not safe. He is not safe in our house. I cannot live like this anymore. You are gone all the time. You do not see what it's like on a day-to-day basis. He is getting bigger. It's just a matter of time before he is flipping dressers and jumping over the gates blocking the stairs. He is going to get out. He is. We don't have a choice."

He looked at me in utter despair. His breathing was labored. *No . . . no . . . no . . . please don't!* He started to cry. Man tears. So many that I wished I'd never spoken a word of this. I wanted to be home in my ten-year-old sweatpants and my torn Notre Dame T-shirt, pretending everything was fine. I wanted to pretend this morning and this evening had never happened. Autism never happened.

"Don't you think I see? You don't think I hear it in that fucking basement? We can't. We can't afford to move. I've run the numbers every way I can. It is not an option." He spoke through gritted teeth.

"But . . ."

"No. I cannot get us out of this. It's not enough. We bought our houses at the wrong time. We're stuck. There is nothing I can do. Nothing. You think I'm blind!? You think I don't know what's happening in my own house?"

If this is the part of the story where you would like to say, "Too bad, so sad," you are entitled. I realize that in this tragic economy we are lucky he is even working. We are lucky to have a roof over our heads. Neither one of us came from money. We earned every dime of what we have on our own. We've never lived beyond our means. Even with a townhouse we've been unable to sell ("Oh, my God, you will sell it like so fast because it is in the best possible location . . ."), we've managed to stay afloat. Then autism—and the myriad of mysterious illnesses that accompany it that the mainstream doctors claim are unrelated. The conferences, out-of-state doctors, immunologists, neurologists, endocrinologists, gastroenterologists. And the therapists: the physical therapy, developmental therapy, occupational therapy, ABA and VB therapy, speech pathology, social skills workshops. He could make one million or twelve million dollars a year. It still would not be enough. It is never, ever enough. It is impossible to put a price on recovery, because the quest for it is never ending—the damage done is *that* extensive.

Another glass of wine and a martini appeared.

His eyes met mine. "I'm scared, too," he said.

I suddenly felt ashamed and terribly immature. I saw a spread-sheet of our financial standing every month. I knew what we had and what we didn't. What I didn't know was that my husband was at the end of his rope. Dave is a doer and a fixer, not a talker. He quietly, without a lot of fanfare, makes things happen. He has accomplished many amazing things over the course of his lifetime with his very unglamorous strategy of quiet, consistent, sustained effort. His pet peeve is people who talk about starting that business, writing that book, losing the weight, etc., and then do nothing to make any of those things happen.

He can't fix autism. He can't fix Noah. He can't fix me. And at that particular moment, he believed he could not keep his family safe. Fucking bullshit autism. I truly hate that stupid made-up word that describes a bunch of behaviors. A useless, official-sounding "ism" created to cover up the greatest injustice ever perpetrated on mankind. Autism is a cruel, unnecessary medical disease born of the quest for extreme profit. We live in a time when prominent nonprofits and scientific and medical institutions worldwide are hiding their crimes by pretending to look for the truth, while subtly tweaking their message—calling immune system damage *dysfunction*; creating the "hot new field" of immunological science; falsely stating the mitochondrial damage they've caused is "rare" and "underlying," implying the discovery of some genetic anomaly will soon help us identify all these vulnerable children before they are born (then we can catch it ahead of time, before killing them is against the law); spending precious millions pretending to look for the elusive autism gene, telling half-truths by selling a vaccine schedule that has never been tested for efficacy, while handing over material safety data sheets to unsuspecting parents that admit "encephalopathy" as a potential side effect of their product. Encephalopathy is inflammation. Inflammation causes autism *because autism is just a made-up word that describes a bunch of behaviors that no one understands—a bunch of behaviors that mysteriously appear after well-baby visits but are completely unrelated.*

Dave was yelling at autism, not me. I felt my rage building. In addition to taking our son's health, his quality of life, his siblings' quality of life, this insidious iatrogenic disease was sapping my husband's pride. My husband, David Michael Peter Goes, is somebody in this world. He commands and deserves respect. Apparently, autism doesn't give a shit.

Miserable, hateful epidemic, you took my son, now you want my husband, too? Fuck you. Fuck you! *You can't have him, you bastard-prick-son-of-a-bitch!*

"You listen to me right now." I wiped away my tears. "You will *not* put this on your shoulders. You have done more than I could have ever asked or hoped for our family. You are an amazing provider, and you have done the right thing by us over and over again. This is not *your* failure. It's not your fault."

I knew enough to stop talking at that point and let him digest.

The table silence gave way to a painful memory.

Dave was in New York, Liam was napping, and Mads was coloring at the dining room table. While sorting through IEP materials in the living room, it occurred to me that Noah was entirely too quiet. I sprinted up the stairs to do a spot check and found him sitting among shards of glass from a lamp that formerly resided on Mads's bedside table. Somehow, he shattered it in its entirety and sat serenely amidst the detritus, scraping out the internal element of the light bulb with his fingers. The lamp was still plugged in. Panicked at the sight of him, fearing his electrocution, I stepped mindlessly through the glass and yanked him to safety. Sobbing, sure he'd ingested some of it, certain it was in his diaper, convinced he was somehow bleeding internally, I checked him from stem to sternum repeatedly. He had not one scratch. Not a drop of blood. When I returned to the scene to clean up, I counted over thirty separate pieces of ragged glass. Not a single cut on our son. Looking back, I see the serendipitous resurfacing of this memory was metaphorical. Here we were, trapped in this monstrous house, with our vaccine-injured child, negotiating his recovery, fighting with insurance and doctors, haggling over IEPs, trying to create lives for our neurotypical children, inspecting and examining every single element of our existence because now we had to; it was no longer a choice. Our house is not what's dangerous. Autism is what's dangerous. Living in a society that refuses to acknowledge its medical genesis and treatment is dangerous. Denial of the autism epidemic is dangerous. Yet, we live among these sharp, piercing, life-threatening truths on a daily basis, walking among legions of unbelievers who are downright hostile to the scientific and medical reality of autism—and we, too, are unscathed. We could find a way to live amidst the shards right where we were planted.

"I know. I know. But I want to make it better, and right now I can't. Can you understand that? And your talking about it infuriates me because I feel like I am letting you down." Dave snapped me back to the present.

I want to make it better, too. That's what we all want, isn't it? Just make it better. Stop the pain, the violence, the suffering. Get someone besides a handful of research physicians to acknowledge the truth in public so treatment won't be so damned hard to get. Moving wasn't going to fix any of these problems for us. Handling it, going through it . . . that's all we could do. Sustain. Remain. Maintain. Live and love each other moment by moment in an unstable world that tells us chicken pox is more dangerous than having a significant portion of our population in diapers and incapable of crossing the street by their eighteenth birthday.

"Of course! I get it," I said. "I get it completely. And you could never let us down."

We collected ourselves and salvaged the evening; we had a baby-sitter for heaven's sake! We finished our second round of drinks, got a little tipsy, enjoyed our meal, and momentarily forgot the enormity of our day-to-day existence. If there's one thing autism has taught us, it's that we have to let go of the shit as quickly as possible and cling for dear life to the good moments.

We started to let go of autism and freed our minds to catch up on everything else in our lives. Within moments the topic turned to good friends of ours who recently divorced. The wife, a friend of mine from the beginning of time, began an affair with the father of one of her daughter's friends. After twenty years of marriage and three beautiful children, she left her husband and married that man weeks after finalizing her divorce. Dave and I were completely taken aback, given the fact they were really great friends. We saw the edges fraying, but they were *the couple* we went to when we needed help. We admired them, their kids, and the life they'd built together.

"You don't understand," she said when she told me her side of the story. "It wasn't like it is with you and Dave. We didn't have that."

Really? I thought about what people see. What they think they see. The house. The weddings and social occasions where we are dressed up and so bloody grateful to be sitting, dancing, and celebrating the fact that we are out in public together. I'm sure it looks quite magical to a disenchanted mid-lifer. But these little glimpses at the respect and deep love we have for each other were earned. We earned the right to kiss on the dance floor, to be giddy when we are free, to act like kids when there are none clamoring for our attention. This is the reward for not leaving, for not giving up. True romance is a delightful side-effect of sacrifice and commitment.

Autism, for all it has taken away from us, has given us a united, unwavering, and indestructible sense of purpose. Dave and I will fight for our Noah's recovery until we leave this earth. We will make those in power aware of every single solitary sick child who could be helped but is not because of archaic laws that favor pharmaceutical companies over sick children and bogus Supreme Court decisions, like *Breusewitz vs. Wyeth*, that promulgate the propagandized notion of "unavoidably unsafe." We will spend the rest of our lives giving voices to the voiceless, telling the stories of thousands of parents we've met, letting these behemoth companies know they cannot continue doing this to our children! We will work in our own community, helping parents who want to know the truth find it. We will shout at the top of our lungs that there is no such thing as better diagnosis, because the phrase "better diagnosis" itself implies to a naïve and believing public that a medical standard of care exists for autism. There is no universally accepted standard of care for autism. Why? *Because autism is just a word, a word that describes a bunch of behaviors that no one understands—a bunch of behaviors that mysteriously appear after well-baby visits but are completely unrelated.*

The Road to Luv Bug's Peeps

My husband and I agree: This child was loved long before he even set foot on earth. As we stood on the beach that June night and stared at the beautiful full moon, we recounted how lucky our son was to already have so much love buoying him up in life. Tim and I had waited over five years after marrying to start our family. Repeatedly peppered with questions about when little Reillys would start appearing, we finally realized that no "perfect time" to have kids would present itself. My mom broke down in tears when we told her I was pregnant. She didn't think she would live long enough to see my kids. There were so many baby showers to welcome this child that I don't think we even had to set foot in Babies R Us until he was at least a month old. We stood there staring at the bright night sky and remarked that by the next full moon, we would have our son in our arms.

After three days of attempting to induce labor and coax this child into the world, he finally relented and popped out. The doctor in charge of delivery was nowhere to be found, and the room's panic button wasn't working, so the nurse was forced to run out of the room to summon her. The only people in the room when Carson finally shot out were Tim and I. Because of the meconium present in the amniotic fluid, we knew there was a risk of aspiration and were concerned. Quickly, the medical team swooped in and took care of everything.

There is nothing like the feeling of watching the labor and delivery nurses gather around your minutes-old firstborn's bassinet, whispering and pointing. At this point in my life, I was a medical novice in terms of observing the behavior of medical professionals, but this gathering hit my radar. I was thinking he aspirated some meconium or something. It did not seem to be life threatening. Maybe they were just talking about the cluster fuck that occurred during my son's birth. Thirty minutes later, a doctor walked into the room. Not my OB/GYN but a pediatric specialist. She was here to tell me there may be "something" wrong with my baby. They didn't know what, but his head was large, his limbs were shorter than those of typical babies, and his tone was a little floppy. They would gather more information, and my pediatrician would stop by in the morning.

It seemed like the best thing to do was to pretend this visit didn't happen, or that it happened all the time. Perhaps everyone was just being super careful. It was easy to ignore this news. There were new stitches for me, forms to sign, and the news that my husband could not stay in the room overnight with me as originally planned. The maternity ward was filled to capacity, so another mom and I had to share a room. For privacy reasons, our husbands could not stay with us.

Around midnight, I was settled into my double room with another new mom who also had some "bad news" that day. All alone, in the quietness of the night, I could finally replay those words over in my brain: "Something wrong . . . floppy tone . . ." I held this beautiful stranger in my arms, paralyzed by fatigue, fear, and love. Tears did not flow until our pediatrician showed up the next morning with pages freshly printed from the Little People of America website.

Our first trip to the city's Children's Hospital was terrifying. With my son barely two weeks old, my husband and I had not yet mastered the basics of parenthood. In addition to trying to figure out this whole diapering/sleeping thing, my son had

major feeding issues. I remember waiting and waiting and waiting to see the specialist. I really didn't imagine my baby's "firsts"
being Baby's First Worthless Genetics Consult, Baby's First Blood
Draw, Baby's First Bone Scan. They don't have sections in the baby
memory book for those milestones.

At this point, we were staring down the barrel of a dwarfism
diagnosis. Physical signs pointed toward it, and now genetics would
confirm it. One in 40,000 people has the type of dwarfism Carson
was thought to have, achondroplasia. Most of these are born to parents of average stature. I won't lie; we were devastated. But as far as
diagnoses go, achondroplasia isn't necessarily as devastating as many
other things you could learn about your baby's health. Most people
with this type of dwarfism are healthy, happy, mobile people. They
are just different—very obviously, physically, visually different.

Achondroplasia is caused by a spontaneous genetic mutation.
You can't pass it on to your kids unless you have achondroplasia
yourself. It affects primarily the long bones in the body, creating a
disproportionate body shape of shorter arms and legs but a nearly
typical-size torso. Also included in the laundry list of differences are
mid-face and skull differences that lead to larger-sized heads, bowed
foreheads, smaller airways, and very disconcertingly—a smaller
foramen magnum. That's the hole at the base of your skull where
your brain transforms into your brain stem and then your spinal
cord. Deformities of the spinal column (narrowing when the cord
goes through the column as well as the shape of the spine) are also
common. If anyone has watched *Little People, Big World* or seen
the Roloffs on Oprah, I can clear this up quickly. Achondroplasia is
the type of dwarfism the mom and the son, Jeremy, have. The dad
does not have this type of dwarfism.

I don't think I had ever seen a person with dwarfism until I was
pregnant with Carson. I took the train into the city every day for
work. Then pre-pregnancy, I would get a nice twenty-minute walk
to the office. When I was pregnant, however, I was exhausted much
of the time. So instead of taking that twenty-minute walk, I hopped
onto the nearby subway that would plop me out right in front of
my office. Selling papers right outside that train station was a man

with achondroplasia. It was memorable because it was the first time I had ever seen a little person (LP). He was there every single day. I wondered about his life, his health, his friends, what school had been like for him. I pondered him a lot those nine months. When I went back to work after Carson was born, he was gone. I never saw him again.

By the ripe old age of one and a half months, my son had his first diagnosis, achondroplasia, confirmed by very specific genetic markers. It was undeniable. At this point, we were glad we could definitively say, one way or the other, what was happening with our child. We learned, while we were waiting for confirmation of Carson's genetics results that children with achondroplasia will sometimes experience some developmental delays. These delays are generally gross motor related. For some reason, there seems to be very little intellectual curiosity in the medical community as to why kids with this type of dwarfism experience hypotonia (low muscle tone) that leads to the gross motor delays sometimes blamed for other developmental delays that occur. "Oh, they just do. For some it's worse than for others." With that explanation, we were prepared for some type of minor gross motor and developmental delays. We informed everyone who worked with us—doctors, Early Intervention, school—that some developmental delays should be expected and are considered normal for kids with achondroplasia.

The dwarfism community is a wonderful community. The organization Little People of America (LPA) focuses on all folks of short stature, with people with achondroplasia being in the majority. The group has a very active Yahoo! message board system, regional get-togethers, as well as an annual national conference. My husband and I welcomed the health information. The LPA has a very official "welcome packet" that was very positive and filled with resources and tips. In that packet was the first time I had seen the "Welcome to Holland" essay. It clicked with my husband and me. This news for our child was so troubling, but the Holland essay gave us hope—he will still laugh and play and be awesome. He will just look different on the outside. It kind of put this new experience in perspective for us.

In addition to medical information, the LPA organization is focused on social interaction. The get-togethers are generally the one place LPs can mingle and not feel out of place. A lot of LPs meet at these conferences and eventually go on to marry. Even more enjoy just "hooking up." This is very typical conference behavior, and I loved it. I couldn't wait for the girls to fall for my gorgeous boy with the long blond hair and beautiful blue eyes in a few years. Our family attended the national conference when it came to our city the year Carson turned two. My husband, mother, brother, and sister-in-law attended with us. My best friend and another friend volunteered at the conference. It was very heartwarming. People were friendly and welcoming to "the community." At that time, Carson was not walking, talking, or even sitting up on his own. People were very encouraging and calmly supportive. All had their war stories about how long they waited for their child or grandchild to walk. It didn't seem like we were that far off the development curve after all.

Of course, there were other looming issues the doctors and the Internet felt it necessary to warn us about, the worst of which was premature death. About seven percent of babies with achondroplasia die suddenly, mainly due to the compression of the base of the brain through the narrowed opening in the skull. We were told to look for any signs that this could be a problem with our new baby. One of the key signs was sleep apnea. Many parents, especially first-time parents, will recall checking to be sure their baby is breathing. Multiply it by a thousand and you've got my anxiety level.

At around six months, we realized that Carson was actually having periods of apnea. The next few years included a dizzying array of sleep studies, MRIs, x-rays, doctor's appointments, excruciating colds, and illnesses that were made worse by the characteristic small airways that achon kids have. Nothing drained from his sinuses or ears. Those darn Eustachian tubes are even narrower in our smaller-stature kids, and almost any ear fluid turns into a huge infection. Throw in a harrowing seizure, along with double pneumonia, and that describes our first eighteen months. Every morning, this child woke up screaming. He was exhausted. He couldn't breathe. He couldn't get into a deep sleep because if he did, his entire airway would relax and collapse on itself. When he recovered from these illnesses, he was no longer talking. Nobody picked up on this: not Early Intervention, not his preschool, not the pediatrician. When we brought it to their attention, it warranted little more than a knitted brow and a "We'll see how he does after his tonsils and adenoids are removed." We did hearing tests to make sure he wasn't losing his hearing, because it seemed like he wasn't responding the way he used to. As it turned out, he could hear fine. After his tonsils and adenoids were removed at age two and a half, he slept a little better and stopped waking up screaming every morning. That was a gift. But at the exact same time, the teachers at his preschool noticed that he seemed to be "in his own world." He had begun humming and "flapping." Early Intervention wasn't worried, because he "only flapped when he was happy." Yep. They really said that. And I wanted to believe it, so I did. I believed the people who said to "wait to see what happens when he starts to walk." I'd have to wait one more year.

When we started hitting what seemed to be more than minor developmental delays (beyond a few months), we started looking for more answers. We questioned our orthopedist and geneticist at the city's Children's Hospital. We met with a doctor who had the largest dwarfism practice in the Untied States and was a world-renowned neurologist. Convinced Carson's dwarfism was the reason for the delays, we were determined to find physiological reasons for the lack of skills. At three, our son was not walking or talking. From a dwarfism specialist's point of view, his body was doing awesome! He had no compressions in his spine, forum magnum, or spinal column. Everything was in tip-top shape.

Dwarfism masked everything. Had it not existed and you were looking at a child with delayed language at fifteen months of age, loss of language at eighteen months following a seizure, along with major gross motor delays, something *may* have raised a red flag. Maybe. But still the conventional wisdom was telling us to "wait and see." Unfortunately, at that point I was still listening to conventional wisdom. Our goal was to wait until he could walk and see what happened with his language. Everyone was hoping the walking would stimulate language. Even a doctor I really respect in the dwarf-ism arena said to us, "Developmental gains happen on a bell curve, and someone is always outside the norm. Unfortunately, it's your son."

And where was I? Asleep at the wheel, almost literally. Sleep was a huge issue with this child. So I was constantly, severely sleep deprived. Even when we gave up on him sleeping in his own bed and he routinely slept with us, he was waking me up every forty-five to sixty minutes to be soothed. He wanted to move constantly, and he couldn't do so on his own. He was obsessed with television and wanted to watch the same shows over and over. This was pre-DVD days, so we burned out three VCR rewinders. He had certain toys he needed to constantly have with him. He loved to swing and spin. I look back now and wonder, "How could I have missed this?" Denial. He couldn't have autism. He is already dealing with achondroplasia. You can't have two major disabilities, can you? Can you? I also think nobody wanted to be the first person to say anything to us. My husband and I are generally nice people, and our son is adorable. Nobody wants to crush the souls of a nice family. So, for a long time, nobody said anything. And we weren't asking. But there was that voice, as tiny as it was, in the furthest recesses of my brain that said, "What if it is?"

I was still visiting the LPA Yahoo! message board, trading advice with other newly diagnosed families, trying to find another family with a three-year-old who didn't walk or talk. Our family would even attend an occasional event. But little by little, those events didn't make sense for us anymore. Our son couldn't walk or talk or play with their kids. He needed a lot of assistance and didn't like being in one place for too long. It was difficult for us to socialize with the other parents while caring for him. Our paths were becoming less and less similar over time. They talked about T-Ball; we talked about out-of-district placements for preschool. I kept in touch with the parents I connected with individually, but LPA didn't fit us anymore. We lost our community.

One day an assistant teacher at his day care asked, "Why can't Carson talk? What kind of speech impairment is it? I was trying to do some research last night, and I wasn't sure if it was apraxia or something else." What? It had never occurred to me to research this issue outside of the context of achondroplasia. I think a light literally went off in my head.

The shift started. I hopped on the computer that night and stayed there. What had I been thinking? I'd left this in the hands of people who went home at night and didn't give me, my son, or my family so much as a second thought. Why? Why had I done that? I found the Cherab website, www.cherab.org. All signs pointed to apraxia as the general speech issue with which my son was struggling. Every once in a while, a new sound or even an entire word would pop out of his mouth, and we would all get excited. Then we would never hear it again. Or maybe we would hear it, but it would be months later. This website led me to the companion Yahoo! group board childrensapraxia.net. Here, I was introduced to essential fatty acids (EFAs) used in different mixtures (DHA, EPA, etc.) to help feed an apraxic child's brain in order to develop the neurological connections needed for speech. It seemed reasonable. My son had severe stomach issues, resulting in constant constipation. This could indicate some type of malabsorption or maldigestion. It seemed like there were very few side effects of supplementing with fatty acids. It was time to sell my husband on the idea.

My husband, Tim, is a scientist. He deals with cold, hard facts and is wary of "ideas from the Internet." But since this idea had such low risk, he was on board. I found a nice bottle of Nordic Naturals EFA at the health food store, broke open some capsules, and sucked them into a syringe. Sounds simple. But if you are new to biomed, or remember being new to biomed, all these steps seem hugely complicated. I could never remember the ratios for the EFAs. The syringes with the bulbs at the top don't hold the liquid in them the right way. Oil is so hard to clean out of syringes. Oh, and how do you get the capsules open without oil squirting everywhere? I ruined more clothes and cleaned oil off of more kitchen surfaces than I even knew we had. I even cracked my tooth getting oil into that child.

Within six weeks of starting his EFA supplementation, he used the American sign language sign for "more." Tim and I stopped in our tracks and looked at each other. Seriously? Did that just happen? This four and a half years old child had been exposed to sign language since he was fifteen months of age. He had spent almost an entire school year in a program that used sign language alongside spoken language and pictures, and he had never used a sign before without prompting. *Never.* And he continued to sign, not clearly, as he has fine and gross motor issues, but he was attempting to communicate. Tim had even forgotten about the EFAs and was almost in disbelief. I had been hoping against hope, day after oil-drenched day that this would happen.

I was hooked. In addition to the information on the Yahoo! message board, there were moms who were just like me. Looking for answers. Confused. Determined. They were so smart. So kind. I felt like I was home. Finally, I had found people who obsessed over their kids the way I did. This was my new community. Within the next few months, a mom on the apraxia board, who just happened to be an MD, noticed that when she removed vitamin E from her son's EFA cocktail, his articulation plummeted. Long story short, she did a bit of her own research and went out on a limb with the board and suggested that vitamin E supplementation would be beneficial to many of our kids. So I approached my husband again. Vitamin E supplementation had a concern of toxicity attached to it, so we agreed to go low and slow and watch for warning signs. I'd won him over with the EFA results. This time, within two weeks of introduction of vitamin E, my son consciously attempted speech in a consistent manner for the first time in four years. The teachers excitedly ran up to me at pick up and told me to watch: "Carson, what does the sheep say?" "Ba," he said with a grin. "What does the cow say?" "Moo," he said proudly. There was not a dry eye in the house.

On the apraxia board, the MD mom had suggested medical tests for diagnosing certain gastrointestinal or metabolic issues that could hinder the processing of these nutrients we were supplementing. I made an appointment with our pediatrician and printed out the list of tests to take with me. I explained my research, new supplementation, results, and my hypothesis to him. He liked the idea and proceeded to painstakingly look up the codes for the tests and write out prescriptions for them. Then he said something to me that I really respected: He told me that he would write out an order for any test I wanted, but he would be unable to read the results. He wouldn't understand what he was looking at or what it meant. He suggested that I make an appointment with a GI doctor or a metabolic specialist. He suggested the city's Children's Hospital. Disheartened but with a plan, I got on the job the next day.

Because we had insurance that didn't need a referral, I was free to use anybody I wanted. So I went to the swanky Children's Hospital website, found a bunch of GI docs and metabolic specialists, identified a couple I thought would be appropriate, and made the calls. The woman who answered the phone was sweet and could not have been nicer to me. I explained that I wasn't sure if I had the right department, but I had been talking with my pediatrician and he suggested I call. She was very friendly and suggested I start with the GI specialist. Then, if the doctor thought it was warranted, they would refer us over to the metabolic department. I thanked her profusely, explaining that this was kind of confusing to me and it had been sort of a hard week. We had just received confirmation of our son's autism diagnosis. As an aside: Yes, we kind of saw it coming, but just like the dwarfism diagnosis, we hoped against hope that someone will swoop in at the last minute and say, "Oh my gosh—*no*! This is *not* the hopeless autism you hear so much about! This is just a simple splinter," or something like that. All who get the diagnosis remember that day/week, or maybe they were too numb to remember. It's a hard time. There was a "Welcome" brochure that came with the autism diagnosis, too. But it wasn't positive; it did not list resources. It had words like "institutionalize," "no known cause," "no cure." It did not have the "Welcome to Holland" essay. Autism is not Holland. Autism *and* achondroplasia—where is that? Zimbabwe? Mars?

So it was lovely to have this very confusing maze of medical mumbo jumbo cleared up by this nice lady making the appointment for me. But when I uttered the last sentence, "We just got our son's autism diagnosis," she changed her tune. "Oh, honey," she said, "we don't treat autism here." "Oh you don't understand," I said, "I'm not asking you to treat his autism. I'd like help with his chronic constipation and malabsorption." "I'm sorry," she continued. "We don't treat autism." I hung up. I was stunned. I was ashamed that I hadn't argued more with her, but have since come to realize two things. First: You probably don't want to fight to be treated in a medical establishment that doesn't want you. Second: She probably saved my son's life.

Again, I went back to my new community—my moms. This was a group of women with kids who had speech problems ranging from inaccurate articulation to being completely nonverbal. Many of us were wondering about autism or already had an ASD diagnosis. There were no other LPs on the board. But back on my LP board, there were moms concerned about speech and developmental delays. They were getting the same advice I had received: "Wait and see." I couldn't stand it. I had to speak up. I had to remove the cloak of dwarfism and force them (and the LP doctors) to view these kids regardless of their stature and consider the possibility of other developmental delays. I was not very popular for that crusade. By now, I had found an autism Yahoo! board that I liked. There are plenty, but this particular board fit my personality. Through this group, I found a list of DAN! (Defeat Autism Now!) practitioners in my state. There were even two who were MDs, which was crucial for Tim and me to feel comfortable with the next phase of this journey.

My son was probably close to six years old by the time he had his first DAN! appointment. Six. So much wasted time. Valuable time. It's that key window of time by which "they" tell you progress or speech or healing is critical. "They" say if you don't see progress by this time, you're not ever going to see it. I would see moms on the message boards who were already treating their sons and daughters before their second birthdays. How I wish I hadn't listened to "wait and see" and had looked past the achondroplasia to see what was really happening to my son. One of the saddest days of my life was my son's fifth birthday party. "They" say that if your child isn't speaking by five, it is likely he or she won't ever speak. Here it was his fifth birthday, and he couldn't speak, couldn't hold a fork on his own, didn't like the texture of cake, and wasn't strong enough to rip the wrapping paper off gifts. It is highly doubtful he even understood the meaning of birthday gifts. But I've learned a big lesson since that day: "They" are guessing.

The more I researched, the more I became convinced that recovery from the myriad of medical problems that present themselves as autism is possible. Recovery is possible. There are children walking around who had autism but don't have autism anymore. I wanted that. I wanted that now. I longed to see my son's personality shine. I wanted him back. I wanted to see him laugh and have fun. I wanted to hear his thoughts and desires. I was heartened that at the root of this idea of recovery was science. Recovery can be controversial to some. "False hope" equals "danger" to them. I think that "no hope" is even more dangerous. How is it acceptable to refuse treatment for a child with excruciating bowel pain? It's not. To deny a child in pain medical interventions would be unethical or, at the least, cruel—unless that child has autism, because in the medical world, it is very typical for children with autism to have bowel issues. According to much of the medical establishment, there is no hope for them. So they get sicker and sicker. By doing nothing, all hope is lost. That is where the true danger lies. The one thing that was unmistakable with our experience was that as my son's bowel issues improved, his mind came back. For us, his bowel is the barometer of his health.

It is four years after my son's first DAN! appointment, and I have my son back. He does not fit into the "recovered" category, but he is recovering. I have always dreamed of knowing my son's thoughts. When communication truly started happening, it was magical and memorable. I'll never forget the night I was snuggling with him and, after verbally reviewing the day's fun activities, I asked him what his favorite part of the day was. I held my breath, afraid he would become frustrated and melt down or simply shut down. He looked at me, signed, and tried to say "elevator." Woo hoo! Or the time he opened his PECS binder at home and pointed to pictures, explaining to us that the lady in the main office of his school had a TV in the phone on her desk (part of the security system for letting people in the building). Or recently, when he got off the school van and said, "Guess what? Alison is going to a different school now." Did my son just say "Guess what?" Gone are the orange crackers with peanut butter that he was obsessed with for years, replaced by carrots and almonds for snacks. Gone are the daily rectal suppositories because he couldn't move his own stools, replaced by sitting on the potty and pooping. Daily. On his own. No diapers. No pull-ups! For us, recovery has come in an ever-changing mix of medical, alternative, behavioral, and social therapies. My "Mommies," as Tim calls them, help me decipher a new set of symptoms or a new therapeutic option. Several of my medical practitioners ask me to consult the Mommies or even defer to them. We are motivated to cut through the crap and look at the science, the results. Don't ever underestimate our power, because it is fueled by one thing—love.

Recovery from dwarfism is not really possible. There are procedures to lengthen bones that will help people with achondroplasia gain height and length on their arms. Of course, this is controversial, at best, within the LP community. I really feel for the people who go through with these procedures. They want what is best for their kids, and then they are left without a "community." They aren't really average stature. For the most part, they still look different. To make matters worse, the LP community almost roundly rejects them, in part because the LP community feels rejected by the person who has the limb-lengthening surgery. A person without a community—we understood that. Our family did not fit into the social network of the LP community with our nonverbal son, who had little to no play skills. Our fit into the autism community was tenuous, too. At social skills groups, Carson was the smallest, weakest child. He looked like he was three when he was eight years old. He had to be protected from his peers. He was unsure on his feet and had little to no peripheral vision. He was weak and slow. The social skills games focused either on verbal skills or on physical activity. If he could participate in the games, it was almost impossible for him to even feel successful, let alone "win."

Don't get me wrong; there are advantages to having a child with autism who also has dwarfism. When he had head-banging meltdowns at the H&M department store, the security guard still looked at me funny, but everyone assumed his meltdowns were of the terrible-twos variety, given his size, instead of a "bad-parenting-of-a-six-year-old"-type tantrum. And when he was given to running away from me when he was angry, I could easily catch him and throw him over my shoulder. I really couldn't imagine how the moms of older, average-stature ASD kids dealt with these issues.

Because every child with autism is so different than every other child with autism, it doesn't seem to matter to autism moms or dads what the differences are. It seems we find similarities or connections. We look for things to bind us together. The parents I've met on this autism journey have been instrumental to my son's recovery process as well as to my own mental health. Autism is isolating in countless ways. Local support groups didn't work for me, because I could never leave the house at night on a regular basis due to my son's high needs. The Internet—the Yahoo! boards and then Facebook—have created communities that not only helped our children but fed our souls and gave us far too many ways to joke about poop.

What happens when I recover my son? What happens when I remove his shield of autism? You know, the shield that keeps him safely unaware of the stares from the young and the old, that keeps him safe from the comments, from the lack of play dates. Yes, it will be wonderful that he will be independent, learning, and healthy. But will he be happy? With the foggy shield of his autism removed, he will realize he is different. He is little, and that really makes a difference to people. They laugh or stare. Girls don't pay attention to him, at least not in *that* way. There will be all these new insecurities that he will have, and maybe he will be pissed. Maybe. Maybe he'll be pissed I took away his shield during the process of his autism recovery. In reality, I embrace this fear as my goal. I'll know I "made it" if this anger erupts. I work toward it every day. When this anger comes, I'll turn back to my LPA community for their help. And my autism Mommies will cheer me on.

PRIMA'S PAS DE DEUX

I remember listening to Tchaikovsky's *Swan Lake*, closing my eyes and dreaming that I was that princess turned into a swan. In those days, all my aspirations revolved around fulfilling that daydream: traveling around the world and dancing one of the most famous pas de deux . . .

Years later, I found myself in an audition room filled with young hopeful ballerinas in the making, filled with the same fire, waiting to hear if I had been chosen to attend one of the city's finest dance schools; then came the positive answer and the burst of joy. My mom, who had traveled from home to help me, taught me all the basics, starting with cooking and paying bills. It was quite a distance from the sheltered family life I was accustomed to, but I knew it was the start of an exciting new chapter of my life. I was discovering North America, going to university, and learning English by watching TV shows—that I didn't understand for the most part! I was living my dream of getting an education and becoming a dancer.

Unfortunately, the dream was short-lived, as only a few years later an injury put an end to the idea of dancing professionally. But I still hoped that one day I might open a dance school and share my love of music and dance with young children. Fortunately, I met my husband soon after and embarked on another beautiful chapter of my life, once again making plans for the future. Life doesn't always turn out the way we plan. Nothing I planned for my son went quite the way I was hoping, starting with the pregnancy.

Having a child was not as easy as I expected it to be, and as I tried one thing after another to get pregnant, longing became obsession. I was determined to do whatever it took, from overcoming my fear of needles to jumping on whatever miraculous treatment or concoction I could find. It was one gigantic roller-coaster ride. As always, my family was very supportive and involved in the early days of my fertility journey. There was no escaping my mother's infamous Moroccan spice mixture, which tasted awful but no worse than the infusions of Chinese herbs, which tasted of gluey tar. At one point, I even traveled to see a healer in Spain, who gave me a special cocktail of pills made out of fish placenta and eggs. I took those pills for weeks on end only to get a full-blown acne reaction and still nothing on the baby front.

For a year I worked with an acupuncturist who repeatedly told me there was a "void" in me that had probably been caused by the death of my beloved younger brother at the age of twenty-six. I put myself through five failed artificial inseminations. Meanwhile, the medical establishment was adamant that there was nothing wrong with either of us. Puzzled doctors told us we were in the gray zone: infertility without a known medical cause. We were devastated.

I no longer attended birthday parties, because I wanted to avoid the looks and invasive questions about why we didn't have a baby yet. I was failing at the most important role of my life—motherhood—and I didn't need to be constantly reminded of it. After years of struggling with my disappointed quest, I decided to take a break from it all. We had lost all perspective on life when all that mattered was getting pregnant. My husband and I had forgotten how to simply go out, have fun, and enjoy life.

A couple of months passed, and my sister-in-law told me about this amazing woman: You would confide your life story, and she would recommend a remedy to fix your problem. I later discovered that she practiced homeopathy, but back then she was just another woman with a miracle solution. The timing was perfect: I was waiting for my second in vitro fertilization attempt, and I was so desperate that I was willing to try anything. After listening to my story, she gave me a remedy. For two months, I did nothing but cry and pray. An overwhelming feeling of grief built up from my brother's death, my inability to become pregnant, and having to give up my childhood dream of dancing. That remedy released all the emotions that I had been suppressing; it was like years of therapy.

Shortly after, I noticed that I was a few days late. The next few days were a torment as I swung between irritability and fear, and excitement and hope. As each day passed, the hope grew: Maybe—just maybe—this was going to be it! On the fifth day, when I couldn't wait any longer, I bought a pregnancy test. I decided that if it was positive, I would figure out a way to surprise my husband.

Over the years, I had waited the nerve-wracking five minutes for a pregnancy test reading countless times with no success, but this time I was late, and it had to mean something. Imagine a woman who has been trying to get pregnant for five years—and who has never been even half a day late in her life—being five days late! When the plus sign appeared, quickly and definitively, I kept opening and closing my eyes to make sure I was reading it correctly. I was shaking and dancing around the house. I couldn't think straight. How was I going to tell my husband?

That night, he came home late to find a little gift box under his pillow with the test in it. When he opened it, we cried, laughed, and looked at each other as if the world had suddenly become perfect. From that moment on, I prayed every day, asking God to protect my baby. I gave up guilty pleasures, watched what I ate, exercised, and refused to go on a plane. I went to all my doctor appointments and ultrasounds. I took first aid classes. My baby was vulnerable, and I was determined to protect him and make sure he was coming into a safe world.

From day one, my beautiful 8.4 lb. boy amazed everyone with his perfect little face and beautiful smile. Even the nurses at the hospital made it a point to pass by and say, "He's going to break some hearts!" My parents didn't arrive until the following morning and were very disappointed to have missed the birth. However, the birth of their first grandchild gave them a renewed interest in a life that had lost all its color since my brother's untimely passing. They never imagined, holding my son for the first time, that they would soon get another slap in the face.

It seemed impossible that anything could go wrong after all my husband and I had gone through in order to have this baby. After five long, heartbreaking years of struggling with infertility, we had had enough challenges. I had suffered so much pain and sadness in my life that surely God was going to give me a well-deserved break.

I had no idea there was anything wrong until D was two and a half. Up until then, I was blinded by the mere miracle of his being here; how could anything possibly be wrong with him? And, as he was my first child, I had no point of reference.

Looking back, I have only vague memories of what happened after he received his first rounds of vaccines. I didn't pay attention, because like most parents, I didn't question his doctor. I took my son to the pediatrician to get his shots without even thinking about their safety. Everything seemed fine until he received his first round of the MMR vaccine. The following week, we went to visit friends in Florida and, as soon as we arrived, D spiked a very high fever that lasted a week. We spent most of that week in the emergency room. Tests were performed but yielded no conclusive answers. Doctors couldn't figure out what was happening. They told us it was a "viral fever." When the fever finally went down, my son woke up a different person. He would run endlessly in circles, making this weird humming sound that we had never heard before. He ran around our living room table for hours on end. At the time, I just thought he had a lot of energy.

The fact that D began talking at the age of two also threw us off. Even if I had suspected that something was wrong, the fact that he could speak surely meant he was fine. He could count from one to ten forward and backward, could name over 200 illustration cards, and could sing any melody from any TV show; he just did not say mummy or daddy. I remember trying to explain things to him, and every time, I got this weird feeling that he did not understand me, as if I spoke a different language. When I think back, I often ask myself, "How could I have been so blind?"

Then one day, I took him to a birthday party. He kept running around the table while I ran after him. All the other moms were having their coffee while their kids socialized. One of the moms approached me and told me that I should have my son evaluated. I stood there in shock and just stared at her. On the way home, I got a sharp pain in my chest and wondered if it was a heart attack. I was having a panic attack for the first time in my life. Pandora's box had been opened, and no matter how much I tried to close it again, it was too late. I remember waking up in the middle of the night in a cold sweat, panic-stricken, with my heart racing so fast that I couldn't breathe. I felt like someone was choking me. I would repeat to myself, "No, no! This can't be happening; he's my miracle baby; he's going to be OK!" I remember thinking, *He is so affectionate and calm; he listens and smiles. All this must be a coincidence.*

It's the worst feeling in the world when you know something isn't right and you can't get yourself to do anything about it. Instead, you avoid it and hope it will go away on its own. I couldn't find the strength within me to make the appointment to have D evaluated. I kept falling deeper into depression and had recurrent panic attacks as my suspicions grew day by day. To calm myself, I sometimes lit a candle in the middle of the night and prayed. It made me feel like I had someone else to confide in besides my husband. It was the only thing that would make me feel somewhat better. I also remember calling my parents and crying endlessly on the phone, leaving them feeling completely powerless and sad.

I think the most difficult part was—and is—seeing my friends' kids develop their abilities to talk, socialize, empathize, express their feelings, and resolve their issues, all seemingly effortlessly, while my son was just not evolving. The gap grew deeper and wider, and all I wanted to do was go into hiding with him. I noticed that the phone rang less often. Kids did not invite him for birthdays or play dates, and I knew I couldn't invite them, because that would force me to publicly expose "our secret." I felt ashamed and hurt, and I found myself once again in the same situation as when I was try-ing to have this child. As much as I did not want to be the center of attention, I was. Every day, I would go to the day care he was attending and avoid talking with the other moms. I would even pick him up early just so I didn't see anyone. I stopped calling my friends, going out, and allowing myself to have fun. I was in the loneliest, scariest place I had ever been in my life. The only person by my side was my husband, who had to be strong because he knew I needed him.

It took me a whole year to make the appointment for the evaluation, and the wait for the appointment was a year and a half. It was the longest, most excruciating year and a half of my life. I would be hoping every morning that my son was going to wake up and be okay. I felt powerless, scared, lonely, and paralyzed with fear. Were hope, willpower, and determination gone forever?

There are days when I think I will never forgive myself for not reacting sooner, but I am slowly learning to forgive myself. I am angry that I did not listen to that little voice in my head, the one that tells you something is not right. Other than that courageous mom at the birthday party, everyone pretended everything was fine and looked away. Our friends and family did not want to hurt our feelings and didn't know how to approach us. The truth is, I wish they had. I wish I hadn't listened to all the "wait and sees." As I watch my daughter grow, I know that if D had been a second child, I would have known much earlier that something was wrong. Maybe then we would have avoided the coup de grace: the second MMR he got while still on antibiotics.

D was finally evaluated in March 2008. I remember sitting behind that glass window, nine months pregnant with my second child (That pregnancy came as a surprise. Of course we wanted a second child but were too absorbed with D's situation to do anything about it. When I look back, I think that unexpected pregnancy reignited the hope and strength necessary to do whatever it took to help our son), feeling numb while my son was being evaluated. I didn't know whether I wanted to cry, scream, or run away. I kept thinking, *This can't be happening. This can't be happening.* I left the hospital that day with the words "no cure," "early intervention," and "small window of opportunity" resounding in my head.

My son was four years old, and I had wasted enough time. That day was my wake-up call; nothing would ever be the same.

I got into solutions mode. I needed information, and I needed it fast; the clock was ticking. I had no time to stay home and hibernate with my newborn. With my mother by my side and my two-week-old little girl bundled in her car seat, I began my race from one therapy center to the next. I was on a mission to find a way to fix my boy.

A friend whose son had speech issues told me about a music therapy center near her. Apparently, this therapy resulted in little miracles for many families, and miracle was definitely the magic word. So, without hesitation, we decided to try this music therapy. It was the first step I took towards my son's recovery, and for the first time in a long time, I felt better. I was finally doing something about the situation, and it gave me unbelievable strength. What we saw that summer blew us away and gave us the drive to go on. D became more aware of his surroundings and started pointing at things and naming them. It was as if he'd opened his eyes for the very first time and discovered the world. I wanted—I needed—more. Those "wow" moments are like a drug; once you get one, you need many, many more.

Unfortunately, children don't come with an instruction manual. I didn't understand why D walked on his tiptoes or ran around the dining room table for hours on end. I couldn't comprehend why, when I called his name a thousand times, he would not answer me, or why, when I talked to him, he would not look me in the eyes. I had to get a better grasp on what was happening. Consequently, my investigation as "Dr. Google" was launched. I spent long hours researching on the Internet. I needed to educate myself and find a doctor. I soon realized that all the biomedical options were in the United States, an unfortunate inconvenience as we live in Canada. My research indicated that MB12 shots might be great for D, so I decided to make an appointment with a biomedical doctor who was known for his MB12 protocol.

The more I read, the more I discovered there was a whole world out there that I had no idea existed. I was full of hope and anticipation. I devoured one biomedical book after another. I was so excited about what these treatments offered that I wanted to share it with the whole world. For the first time, animated by hope, I started to open up about what was happening to us. When I talked to my family about the treatments, the ones we were doing or wanted to do, people noticed that the fire in my eyes was back— and I intended it to stay!

I wanted to start everything right away: the diet, the methyl B12 shots, and the supplements. Now that I knew there were things I could do to reverse the damage and save my son, his recovery became my full-time job. It was the first thing on my mind when I woke up and the last thing on my mind before falling asleep. I wanted to learn everything that had worked for others. I was hungry for success stories; they fueled and inspired me. Why not try everything? I had already fought a battle to get this baby, how could I not fight another to get him healthy? I kept thinking, "If other kids can do it, so can we!"

Through this entire journey, I have been blessed with the most amazing and supportive partner. When we were trying to have a baby, my husband encouraged me to try everything as long as it was safe. Even in our darkest hours he always believed in us and that we would have a family. His faith is unshakable. I often wish I were more like him. He's been holding my hand ever since that day in March 2008, and he's never let go. He made sure I didn't fall apart, because he knew that both our son and our yet-to-be-born daughter needed me to stay strong. To this day, whenever the road gets difficult and bumpy, he is the one who reminds me to never give up.

Through Yahoo! support groups, I discovered many other parents were eager to learn and share their experience. I finally felt like I wasn't alone anymore. I realized that hundreds of other parents from all over the world were going through similar, and sometimes even worse, situations. That's how I met Money, one of my coauthors. We had the same doctor and often exchanged ideas on the doc's Yahoo! support group. I remember posting questions and hoping that either Money or another mom, who had brought her son back to full health, would answer me. They both inspired me with their profound knowledge. I wanted to become as knowledgeable as they were so that my son could get better as fast as possible. I did not have a minute to waste, so I would flood them with questions about enzymes, probiotics, vitamins, minerals, diets, HBOT, methylation pathways, mitochondria disorders, PANDAS, antivirals, antibiotics, antifungals, and more. This group brought me a certain level of comfort. The more options I knew about and implemented to improve my son's diet, health, and environment, the better and stronger I felt. So did he.

Simultaneously, I was discovering the unique rhythm of our mother-and-son pas de deux. Healing my son was not a simple exercise: one step forward, two steps back, all while trying to keep our balance and a steady tempo. There were good weeks and bad weeks. There were moments of immense joy and moments of complete despair. There were many sleepless nights and lots of obstacles in the midst of all the little victories. Still, I continuously pushed my family to move on to the next step. Once we established the new diet, we needed to implement the methyl B12 shots and vitamins. After we had those in place, we purchased a mild hyperbaric oxygen therapy (mHBOT) chamber. Step by step, we worked together toward reaching our next goal.

We learned that D had pediatric autoimmune neuropsychiatric disorder associated with streptococcal infections (PANDAS), and we could not seem to find an appropriate treatment. Feeling somewhat desperate, I emailed Money. I needed to talk to someone because I was at a crossroads and didn't know what to do anymore. My instincts drew me to her because I sensed a tremendous kindness and humanity in her posts. A mom in the PANDAS group was getting amazing results thanks to homeopathy. It turned out Money was also into homeopathy and was getting very encouraging results. She suggested I read *The Impossible Cure*, by Amy Lansky, and gave me the contact information for her own homeopath. In my most desperate hours trying to conceive D, I had turned to homeopathy. It seemed we had come full circle. I took it as a sign that this was the next step to take on our path to healing him.

A month later, remedy in hand, we began the next phase of D's recovery road. And I am so glad we did! Money and I have become good friends. We speak regularly on the phone, and I know one day—sooner rather than later—we will meet in person. She invited me to join a group of strong, smart, devoted parents that became the Thinking Moms (where I was nicknamed Prima, in reference to my past as a dancer).

This group is like nothing I had ever experienced! We share our knowledge (biomed, homeopathy, and pretty much everything else) and the details of our kids' journeys toward recovery. We cry; we scream with joy. We are our true selves, and it feels so good. We have become very close and care deeply about one another. Every day, I enjoy breakfast with the Thinking Moms while sitting at my computer, coffee cup in hand. They taught me English slang and the art of writing a post. But most of all, they taught me the true meaning of hope and perseverance. Some of the moms have succeeded in restoring their kids' health, giving them the opportunity to attend a mainstream classroom and develop friendships. Some, like us, are well on their way to recovery.

As I reflect on the past year, my mind wanders, and I find myself forgetting to look back. I'm spontaneously thinking forward. This year was a good year: D made huge strides. He discovered his baby sister. He's insatiably curious about the world he lives in. He asks questions about everyone and everything, as if all this time he'd been behind locked doors. In light of all his progress, focusing on the future comes naturally. The momentum is so great, the ride so thrilling, that there seems to be no need to look back. I am filled with anticipation and excitement about what will come next for him. He is nothing short of amazing, and he is, along with all our kids, a real hero.

I am slowly allowing myself to live and love again. I want to help others and share what this journey has taught me. I feel compassion for other parents who are just entering this scary, mind-spinning black hole. I want to hold their hands and tell them it's going to be all right. It took time, but today I am grateful for everything that has happened to me. It has made me a better and stronger person. Who would have thought that I would be sitting here one day, writing a chapter about the most painful period of my life with peace in my heart and faith in the future?

I realize now that I have been dancing the most important role of my career: a pas de deux with life, but more importantly, a pas de deux with my son. For the first time in years, I am dreaming about dancing again, but this time I want it to be with my kids—all of our kids—holding their hands and showing them the beauty of music and rhythm. I want to tell them that they can fly and the sky is indeed the limit. Who knows? Maybe my childhood dream of becoming a dancer will come true, only this time it will have a deeper and more meaningful purpose than I ever imagined.

B.K. Lets Go of the Controls and Holds Tight to Faith

I can do all things through Him who strengthens me.
—Phillipians 4:13

You never think it is going to happen to you. As little girls growing up, we tend to imagine what life will be like when we grow up. We will marry a romantic man, have a big wedding in a palace; have six beautiful, perfect children, live in a gigantic house in the suburbs, and be filthy stinkin' rich. Of course, it varies a little with each individual girl's fantasy, but in essence it's all the same. We dream of having an ideal life, and we don't imagine that it could be any other way. When we grow up, it's all supposed to be perfect. It never is. And for some of us, it's less perfect than it is for others.

When L. C. was born, I thought he was absolutely perfect. Never mind the fact that he was a "he" when I had dreamed all my life of having a house full of little girls. After all, I had grown up in a house with three older brothers. I was destined to have a daughter; God wouldn't let me down! But it didn't take long after seeing that first ultrasound image to completely fall in love with the son that God knew I needed and who needed me. Childbirth was full of all the modern amenities: Pitocin, antibiotics (strep B mom here), epidural, you name it, that all culminated in a C-section. He was such an amazing gift! I was a careful new mom. I did everything I was told to do. If the American Academy of Pediatrics said to do it, I did it. So, of course, I vaccinated my son up to his eyeballs. He received his first vaccination at less than twelve hours old, before his immune system even had time to wake up. Giving a hepatitis B vaccine to a newborn? Of course! Whatever the doctors said! I didn't do any research; I didn't ask any questions. I simply trusted the doctors to know what was best.

As L. C. grew, even during his first year of life, month by month, it became increasingly apparent that he was different. "Quirky" was how I used to describe him. He sat up, rolled over, crawled, and walked all on schedule. He just didn't talk. He also didn't seem to like attention. Whenever we would applaud him for completing a new task, he would sob brokenheartedly. As a new mom with a "perfect" baby, I simply embraced his quirks and listened to his pediatrician when he told me that some boys were just late to talk. Meanwhile, the autism warning signs blared all around me. He hated loud noises and detested strangers. He could ignore you as though you didn't even exist. Finally, before his second birthday, I started my Internet research and figured out that he had autism. There was no question about it; he had many of the signs. When my husband got home from work one night, I sobbed my discovery to him. He got angry with me for even suggesting that something was wrong. He remained locked in his denial for years. I allowed him that. In fact, I actually followed suit, praying that I was wrong and my husband was right.

I have to admit, I didn't worry much about L. C. He was such a good boy. I always referred to him as my little "shopping buddy."

He gladly went with me everywhere I went. He was very well behaved and quiet. Unlike many kids with autism, he accepted my affection and had no difficulties transitioning into new situations. For me, that just made it easier to accept him as simply quirky. The only real obvious problem was his lack of speech. I thought that he was so bright that speech would eventually come. I thought that because he was so easygoing, autism wasn't a real problem, at least not for us. It would all get better. I just knew it.

Locked in my denial, I continued to be a good mommy and followed the doctor's orders. I continued vaccinating and never considered that to be a problem.

That all changed shortly after his fifth birthday.

L. C. had developed a chronic stuffy, runny nose. It lasted for months. We took him to an allergist who ran all of the run-of-the-mill allergy tests and, with the exception of peanut and penicillin allergies that had been discovered years before, he was proclaimed to be allergy-free. The allergist declared that "viruses" were the cause of his chronic congestion. We took L. C. back to the same pediatrician who had already put him through two rounds of antibiotics that season. The pediatrician put him on yet a third round of antibiotics. It was the third round in about four months. That's when everything changed.

My sweet, easygoing, loving little boy changed right before my eyes. The most alarming thing: He started banging his head on the floor. *Hard.* He would scream loudly and throw himself on the floor, slamming his head so hard that he bruised it. It would happen seven or eight times a day. It was the most difficult thing in the world to watch.

Back to the doctors we went. We had him tested genetically. He went through an MRI and a multitude of other tests. All came back normal. No one had any answers as to why this was suddenly happening. Truthfully, no one could even agree on autism as a diagnosis either. One examiner said it kind of looked like autism and that autism was the best diagnosis he had, though it didn't exactly fit. L. C. was interested in people and affectionate with mommy, and that perplexed the examiner. The examiner also applauded our decision to homeschool L. C., because he felt it likely that our son would need to be restrained in a school situation.

The geneticist didn't believe it was autism at all. We were told to get a behaviorist to help with the head banging. But behaviorists aren't covered by insurance, and with me being a stay-at-home mom, we didn't have the luxury of paying for the high-priced therapies commonly used to treat autism. As L. C.'s mom, I honestly knew in my heart that a behaviorist couldn't help him. We had to find the root of the problem.

One night, during a head-banging episode, I believe God let me in on what was happening. It was as clear as if He had spoken to me audibly and shined a light on my son, who was in distress, screaming and banging his head. I finally recognized the truth: This was not a behavioral issue; this was a physical illness. Head banging was L. C.'s response to pain.

Just the day before this revelation, I had heard about the gluten-free, casein-free (GFCF) diet. That was no coincidence. That night, after realizing that L. C.'s head banging was a pain issue, I talked to my husband at length. We decided that we would try the GFCF diet for a few days and see what happened. What happened seemed like a miracle! Within two days L. C.'s head banging dramatically diminished, and his demeanor completely changed. He was happy, sweet, and interactive again.

We found a doctor nearby who was trained in treating kids with autism using diet and supplements. He also took insurance! It was this doctor who finally helped my husband and me see the connection between vaccines and autism. You see, there are factors to look at before vaccinating that can help you determine if your child is at a higher risk for autism. If you or your spouse have allergies, asthma, autoimmune disease, or diabetes, then your child is at risk of having a compromised immune system. If your child's immune system is weak, his body will be less likely to be able to remove the toxins from the vaccines. My husband has suffered from horrible allergies his entire life, and I suffered from an autoimmune disease before I got pregnant. If the medical community would finally admit the connection, there would be a way to determine which kids were at higher risk of developing autism. It might not work in every case, but I know in our case we could have seen this coming. We, as a society, are being repeatedly lied to about the vaccine-autism connection. I know this. I am as confident that this connection exists as I am about the sun shining today. Without a doubt, I believe it is true.

The GFCF diet is not a cure. While I wish I could say that L. C. never had any more head banging, I can't. It rears its ugly head from time to time, depending on his state of health. The vaccinations and antibiotics have destroyed his gut, so we have to remain vigilant. Over the years, I have learned how to manage the head banging with diet and supplements. When he does have an occasional episode, I almost always know exactly what he needs in order to stop it. I have come to believe that L. C.'s condition is caused by a toxic overload, and we have to keep that toxic load to a minimum in order to keep him feeling well. It requires frequent interventions and much trial and error. But once I learned about diet and supplementation, it made his symptoms much more manageable, and in turn, L. C. started doing much better.

After managing L. C.'s symptoms for two years, we decided that for the long-term benefit, we would try Andy Cutler's chelation protocol. It involves using chelators at very low doses in frequent intervals to safely remove heavy metals from the body. L. C. had tested positive for lead, and we thought mercury was probably also lurking in his body. Cutler's chelation takes years to complete, but it has a very high success rate. After doing this chelation under a doctor's supervision for a while, we started seeing some very promising and exciting improvements.

Unfortunately, in February 2010, another crisis hit our family. I was diagnosed with breast cancer. Not only did I have breast cancer but it had metastasized to a small area of my pelvic bone.

Boy, my life had *really* strayed away from my childhood fantasies! I began chemotherapy right away, followed by a lumpectomy and then radiation. While I know these therapies are not ideal, after much prayer I decided that this was the direction of treatment that I needed to pursue. All the while, I remained vigilant about caring for L. C. and keeping him comfortable and happy. Before you begin feeling sorry for me, let me just say this: This was one of the most blessed periods of my entire life. Up until that point, I was really trying to do it all. I was trying to call all the shots in L. C.'s care, and that was a tremendous burden. I was trying to go through life solely on my own strength, neglecting my Christian faith. My relationship with the Lord was fragile and minimal. When I was diagnosed with cancer, everything changed. I knew I didn't have the strength for this, and I learned that God could use this experience for good. Romans 8:28 says, "And we know that God causes all things to work together for good to those who love God, to those who are called according to His purpose." To gather God's strength, I dug deep into His word, and my relationship with Him flourished. It was through this experience that I learned the most valuable lessons of my whole life, and I have watched in amazement how He has worked in my life. You see, when we let go of control of things in our lives and give them over to God, He takes them from us and does some pretty amazing things. It's very hard to let go! Our nature as humans is to try to be in control. But the truth is that there is very little that we can actually control in life. If we *did* have control, we'd be living those fantasies that we had as kids. When we surrender control to God, He takes our lives and makes them what *He* intended them to be. It might appear you are losing control, but it actually sets you free.

I believe many times God uses trials to draw us closer to Him. It's an amazing thing! People tend to look at me like I am crazy when I say that having breast cancer has been a blessing, but that's truly what it has been. I've fallen in love with Jesus. I've learned to trust that whatever God has in store for me is truly His best, even if I don't understand it. I'm learning to give each decision that I have to make, including the small ones, to Him before I act. It's kept me from making some very bad mistakes, and all the while He is showing me His work in my life. It's awesome to see! God never promises in His Word that life will be easy for His people. In fact, it's quite the contrary. He promises that we will endure trials and hardships. It's how you deal with these trials that helps you grow the most as a follower of Christ.

At the present time, L. C. is doing better. He is nine years old, and he still has autism, but he is functioning at a much higher level than he did even just one year ago. His head banging episodes are much less severe and much less frequent. I'm praying that as time goes on, those episodes will disappear completely. We are focusing on reducing his toxic load, and I believe that is the key to his recovery. In the meantime, he is a sweet, loving little boy who is happy as long as he is feeling well. And keeping him feeling well is my job in life.

I don't know what the future holds for L. C. or me. I pray that I am able to stick around on this planet long enough to see L. C. grow up and be healthy. But truthfully, I don't believe that is for me to worry about. Matthew 6:34 says that we should "not worry about tomorrow, for tomorrow will care for itself. Each day has enough trouble of its own." I need to tape that one to my refrigerator. I have to work on remembering that every single day. But I believe God has a plan and His plan is better than any plan of my own. No, He didn't give my son autism. My son was born healthy. The world gave my son autism. But somehow God can use it. None of it makes sense to me right now, but I do believe that one day it will. I just have to hold on tight to my faith and to my Lord and take life as it comes, one day at a time.

It's still hard sometimes, and I struggle. As a Christian, I don't feel I get as much support from the Christian community as I should. That is probably the most heartbreaking thing. My church holds a "flu shot day" every year, on which members can go into the fellowship hall and get their shot. I'm afraid this year I allowed it to make me feel angry and bitter. The church largely continues to be blinded to the dangers of vaccines and holds great trust in anyone with an MD degree. I know that many think I am crazy because I believe in the vaccine-autism connection. They don't understand me. I can forgive them for that because if it hadn't happened to us, I wouldn't understand it myself. All I can do is keep praying for the Lord to remove their blinders. I pray for that all of the time. In the meantime, I continue to watch their kids suffer from effects that I am now certain are the result of vaccine overload.

I have found such great strength in the autism mom friends that I have met online. One particular group I belong to is especially strong: The Thinking Moms' Revolution (TMR). We all come from different backgrounds, different faiths, and different communities, but we share one important, common bond: We are all moms (and one dad) of children with autism, and we love our children more than we love ourselves. We will sacrifice whatever we have to in order to make our children's lives better. We are so blessed to live in a time that we have easy, instant access to one another for love, support, and advice. I thank God for these friends! I couldn't have made it this far without them! I love each one of them so very much.

Oh, and my TMR nickname B.K.? It stands for Booty Kicker because I'm kicking cancer's *and* autism's booties!

Mama Mac Gets Her Groove Back

You know the expression, "When you've met one child with autism, you've met one child with autism?" It's true about autism parents as well. We arrive at the day of our child's diagnosis having accrued different life experiences, with different levels of resilience, hardened resentments, and varied support networks. We choose different treatment paths for our kids. Some parents become very political. Some lose their marriages and end up caring for their children as single parents. Some parents find a peaceable way forward; others fall into addiction. And a few find no way forward at all and take their own lives, and sometimes the lives of their children with autism as well. We have many differences, but just as our kids share the common thread of autism, we autism parents share the fact that we love our children deeply.

I'm not speaking here about the experiences of my family or, in particular, my son's experience of autism and healing. My sense of myself has changed a lot because of autism, and that is my focus here. My experience as an autism mom is just that, my experience. Some of what I feel may resonate for other parents, and some may sit in stark opposition. I would never dare to assume I speak for anyone else but myself.

I glimpsed autism on the horizon when my son, Nick, was sixteen months old. Nick has a typically developing sister, four years older than he is, so I had a general sense of what development should look like at this stage. After a little over a year of sweet, healthy babyhood, Nick began to look anything but typical. Nick's health and development fell off sharply after his fifteenth month vaccines (DTaP, MMR, and Hib). I was worried but not in a "front of your mind, talk to your husband" kind of way. More like I had a conversation going on in the back of my head all day: "Why is he just spinning the wheels on the toy cars he used to play with?" "Why is he screaming so much?" "When did he suddenly become so unhappy all the time?" "What's up with the yellow, stinky diarrhea?" "Why is he sitting, staring into space?" "When was the last time I heard him speak? My God, I think he's stopped talking!"

One afternoon, when Nick was sixteen months old, I was standing in front of his bureau, putting his sweet baby clothes away, when these worries crashed from the back to the front of my brain. This child was not okay, and I knew it.

At twenty-one months, Nick was formally diagnosed with PDD-NOS. Nick is almost seven years old now. I have not stopped worrying about him, and my anxiety doesn't show any signs of letting up. I've always been a worrier. I worried as a child. My parents told me in fourth grade that I needed to learn how to "stop and smell the roses." I worried as a single woman in my twenties: "Does he like me? Will he call?" I worried in my thirties as a mom prior to autism: "Is this the right nursery school for her?" "Do these jeans make me look fat?" But now as a mom of an autistic child, I have raised worry to an art form. In this, I know I am in good company.

I know I'm also in good company in the devastation that hits with an autism diagnosis. A mom I know told me that for a year after her son was diagnosed, if someone simply asked, "How are you?" she would burst into tears. My coping mechanism was to jump into action and set up services like my hair was on fire. Within two weeks of the diagnosis, we had a full-time behavioral program running out of our home. After all, the developmental pediatrician had made it sound like Nick had always had autism, I had just missed the cues. I have been a psychotherapist for twenty years, but that's not how I knew she was wrong. I knew that he had not been born with autism because I am his mother, and I felt the strong connection between us, and then I felt it fade. But she made it sound like time was everything; we had to try to pull him through that magic window before the age of five. All I could hear in my head now was the sound of an intense little coxswain screaming through a bullhorn, "Ready to row! Power ten!" I did not enjoy having a full-time behavioral program running in my home. Don't get me wrong; the providers were loving, hard-working, terrific young women. I just suffered being immersed and isolated in autism in my home all day, every day.

Nick was diagnosed over the summer. In the fall, I took my daughter back to school and faced the parents of her friends, my friends. I felt like I had crossed an ocean that summer. When school ended in June, I was still on the shore with all the other families untouched by autism. Over that summer, we left them all behind and set sail on this strange and lonely journey. In hindsight, I wish I was the kind of autism parent who was quiet about the diagnosis, sat with it a while, and then chose carefully who to seek support from. Not me. I've always needed to talk through my stuff, and I cried desperately to my friends about what had happened to my sweet Nick. They were patient and loving and kind, but they didn't get it, and that left me feeling more isolated. That was 2006, and I didn't know anyone with a child with autism.

I was a basket case, and I covered it up with a harsh forced smile, which was about as effective as cheap concealer on a nasty pimple. As a defense technique, I tried to beat the other person to questions first. I would ask them, "How was your summer in Nantucket? Must have been lovely," even though I didn't care. There would be no vacations for us now, and the idea of the rest of the world carrying on made me sick. Rarely, someone would squeeze in a "How are you?" or "How is Nick doing?" Everyone knew, by the way. I told the UPS driver, the pharmacist, even the toll collector on the highway, because I was in so much pain. Admittedly, I'm also a bit of a bitch, so there was a flavor of "Hey, you think your life is just ticking along. Well so did I, and then *whammo!* Autism! Just so you know, it could happen to you, too." My forced smile made my face hurt and led to cheerfulness fatigue, and I was fooling no one.

My mom came to stay with us about six months PD (post diagnosis). She walked in the door and said, "Oh my God, honey, you are so depressed." The fact that depression was an appropriate response to the situation was a little lost on her. But the point is, she saw through my veneer. What I saw, if I let my guard down and looked in the mirror, was terror.

In the beginning, I struggled so much with the diagnosis. I did everything I could to present Nick to his neuropsychologists in the best possible light, hoping like crazy he wouldn't qualify for the diagnosis. I still see parents new to autism doing the same thing, and I totally get it. For one evaluation, I let Nick eat an entire bag of parmesan-flavor Goldfish crackers in the car on the way because I wanted him to be full of energy. Oh the irony. He did terribly that day, in part due to the fact that his body couldn't digest wheat or dairy, and those crackers have among the highest levels of MSG (brain glue) found in children's food. They don't call it "baby crack" for nothing.

After the Goldfish crackers incident, my husband bought me Jenny McCarthy's first book about her son, Evan. He might have bought it because she's a knockout, but I'll forgive him for that because it was a complete game changer for me. I finished Jenny's book in one day. I can remember where I was sitting and what I was wearing while I read, in the same way people can tell you exactly where they were when they heard that JFK was shot. That was when it dawned on me that I was right. Nick was very sick. His autism wasn't separate from the physical mess his body had become. His immune system had been overwhelmed and had crashed from too many vaccinations and antibiotics in too short a period of time. Autism was the neurological result of that. This horrible, tragic nightmare could have been prevented. I wanted to lift up the window and scream out to the world. I thought, *My God, we don't have a minute to spare. We need to tell everyone. We need to stop this madness.*

Not one more child should have to go through what Nick has. That night I emptied the kitchen of every bit of food that had gluten or dairy in it, and we began the diet the next day.

My passion to learn as much as I could, as quickly as possible, about what was making Nick so sick led me into lots of Internet chat groups where I was shocked to find I was in tremendous company. And we all had such similar stories. Suddenly, I wasn't so isolated. And the parents were so helpful: reviews of providers, must-read books, supplements to try, dinner recipes for special diets—and compassion. I found great big virtual hugs filled with understanding. I was not alone anymore. It hit me one morning while driving the kids to school that this was life after one of the worst things has happened: The rules don't apply anymore. After all, I had followed all of the rules with Nick, and look where it got me: autism. We would make up new rules. There was a great pioneering sense of freedom that came with this change of heart.

After I started to get my groove on with biomedical treatment for Nick, I began to get in touch with how very angry I was. I felt deeply betrayed by the medical establishment, and I could barely contain my rage that my child had been so seriously hurt, so needlessly. My eyes had a wild glint in them. I was fiery and easily ignited. I channeled my anger by getting politically active with autism. I started commenting on blogs and even started a blog of my own. I made bumper stickers and put flyers with vaccine ingredients on the windshields of parked cars. I was on a mission. I read everything I could find on all sides of the conversation about vaccine safety and autism. I talked to everyone about this and probably drove a good many of my friends crazy. Overnight, I had gone from a bereft mom with a child recently diagnosed with autism to Erin Brockovich. One day, jogging in Cambridge, I ran past a young mom trying to soothe a very fussy baby. The cry was the familiar feral scream that haunted me from Nick's regression. Before I could stop myself, I yelled out to her as I huffed and puffed, "Please stop vaccinating that baby!" As she looked at me, bewildered and irritated, I realized I must have looked absolutely insane. I was zealous, to say the least, and my heart was in the right place, but my delivery was going to need some work.

I started to volunteer as a Rescue Angel for Jenny McCarthy's organization, Generation Rescue, which felt highly gratifying. These were moms who wanted to talk about healing autism and wanted help. This reduced my compulsion to bore every mother on the playground with my vaccine concerns. I joined the ranks of the moderators of our state autism Yahoo! group and began to read *Age of Autism* online every morning before I read the newspaper. I flew down to D.C. and marched in the Green Our Vaccines rally. On that flight, I met another autism mom. She led me to our DAN! doctor, who has made an unbelievably positive difference in my son's health. That's how autism has worked in my life: The more I put myself out there, the more help and support comes back for Nick. I could tell you five more stories like that one. I can also tell you that I hear this same story over and over from other autism parents. We call it "paying it forward," like the movie with Kevin Spacey. I started going to a yearly autism conference in Chicago, and I come home every year feeling simultaneously empowered, exhausted, and thrilled to get moving with new ideas for healing Nick. At the rally, at the conferences, and online, it is clear to me that I am in the most amazing community of parents. I feel connected to brilliant and lovely people who are as deeply passionate about helping their autistic children as I am. It makes some of the ignorant and painful things that are said to me, like, "He's so lucky to have you," or "I don't know how you do it," hurt a little less. At least now I have a good place to talk about them.

I look back at this time, and I wish I could have been a more refined version of myself. I wish I could have held more back, not dumped this conversation on everyone, everywhere. But I couldn't. It's just not my way. I am a highly verbal person. I was in shock, and I did the best I could to take care of myself, which for me meant talking about it. It was chilling to me how little some people seemed to care about this. Many other autism parents I've spoken to have had the same experience. When they figured out what happened to their child, they expected the world to care and to make changes. The world couldn't have cared less. I'm always shocked when I find out about new vaccine injuries in little one- or two-year-olds. Nick is six now, and I have been talking about this loudly for four solid years. How could they have not heard me?

My anger was activating and fired me up, but there were a lot of moments lost in thought on the couch with a blanket over my head, usually after consuming a large amount of chocolate. I have spent a lot of time over the last four years very worried and very sad about autism. I hate the expression "Autism is a marathon, not a sprint," which is frequently doled out as advice to new autism parents. In part, I hate it because it's true. When I initially heard it, I secretly thought, *I'm going to ignore that because if we work hard enough, it won't be a marathon for us, we'll be done with autism.* Yeah, well, I was wrong on that one. It did turn out to be a marathon, and that meant a course correction. You cannot run a marathon solely on adrenaline.

As I meditated under the blanket on how sorry I felt for myself, a powerful idea came forward. It occurred to me that this was my one go-around on this planet, and I could make of this situation what I wanted. I could choose to have a pity party for the next forty years, or I could choose a different outcome. The pity party sounded so martyred and long suffering. I couldn't even stand the idea of being with me. Could I make misery look sexy? This felt a little like having too much fun too close to the death of a loved one. Was it sacrilegious for us, as an autism family, to enjoy ourselves? No, damn it! It was imperative. It wasn't giving in and saying, "Oh, this is all right with us; we're fine." It was probably the only way we were going to survive this. It's like sex between parents of a child with autism. You have to do it because the autism marriage statistics are terrible. It's a political gesture. It is your autism patriotic duty. So legs in the air ladies, and think of England!

It became necessary to address the fact that I looked like shit. Spending all of our money on biomedical care for Nick was not an excuse for the extra thirty pounds of worry weight I was carrying. That would have to go. It made me feel weak. If I'm fat and feeling insecure, the bad guys win again. It was important to me to start feeling physically stronger. I wanted people to listen to me, and I felt like they weren't going to if I were in my baggy sweats. "Autism parents have to take care of themselves" is about as welcome a comment as mentioning that "autism parents should have a regular date night." However true it may be, it is ridiculously hard to pull off. Our kids are sick. As we pursue medical treatment for our kids, many autism parents, especially moms, find out that they are suffering from many of the same ailments as their kids; leaky gut, yeast, thyroid issues, inflammation, or poor ability to detox, among others. It's hard for autism parents to justify the time and money for their own medical care. On the downside, I have seen some autism moms get really sick when they ignore their own health. When you add the endless responsibilities toward kids with autism, the destructive toll constant worry takes on people's health, and these immune system vulnerabilities, it is no wonder. If for no other reason, sometimes I am motivated to take my health seriously because Nick may need me far, far into his adulthood.

As I started to pull myself together, I realized that the closer I came to living the truth about what happened to Nick, the less I needed a smoke screen to keep me from my pain. I think it's easy to rationalize lots of comforting things that do your body no good when you've had your heart broken by autism. The wine, cigarettes, and chocolate in excess keep us a safe distance from our heavy feelings. After a day of listening to nonstop verbal stimming, we feel justified. It's not a great solution, though. For me the smoke screen can be overeating, procrastination, too much Chardonnay, a pack of Camels—I could go on. My truth is: My son was born healthy and regressed into autism after a toxic overload, which included vaccinations. Working to heal him and our family from this trauma, while pursuing honest science and justice for children with autism, is living my life as close to my truth as possible.

It was, and is, an active choice to remain optimistic on this journey. Autism is one of the first things I have encountered in my life that I have not been able to conquer with tremendous effort alone. The outcome is not necessarily dependent on how hard one works. Some children get miraculously better with small interventions.

Some kids can have the whole biomedical panoply thrown at them and still make minimal improvements. It's a crapshoot, literally, in our house. Some days go better than others. I try not to whine too much about autism, but every once in a while, I'll have a good bitch. I have been newly devastated every time we've had neuro-psych testing done. It's always autism. Now I'm just looking for the best strategies to help Nick gain skills and move forward academically and socially. Screw the diagnosis. "It is what it is," as one autism mom I know has on a poster hanging in her dining room.

I think, fundamentally, that moving from a sad, victimized place to one of a survivor has put me in a more energized role as Nick's advocate. I'm no longer walking into IEP meetings full of resignation that he won't get the services he desperately needs. In my "survivor head space," I am also more energized for the tiny little interactions he and I have every day, for instance, when I'm helping him put on his shoes. In the past, I might have sat him on my lap, put the shoes on for him while staring into space and worrying about him as an adult living in a poorly run group home. Now, I am more likely to sit with Nick face to face, trying to teach him how to put the shoes on himself, and we might share a giggle. The spirit of our connection is more present.

Nick is my hero. I consider him to be a very strong and brave little boy. I feel guilty as hell that his life got off to such a rotten start due to shitty medical decisions. People tell me I shouldn't feel guilty, but I do. I just do. But I also feel a tremendous sense of purpose in my life. I was a bit insufferable before autism. I used to be far more interested in what I looked like while I was doing something than whether or not I was genuinely happy. Autism has given me humility and wisdom, and I am grateful for that. I no longer sweat the small stuff, and I pity people who fall apart over what I consider luxury problems. Autism has led me to some of the coolest people I have ever met. I shudder sometimes at the thought that without Nick's vaccine injury and subsequent autism, I might never have crossed paths with many of these parents. Although I wish I could have toned myself down a bit in the earliest days of Nick's diagnosis, there has been an upside to being so "out there." I'm included in lots of conversations about potential therapies or providers to try, and the community of love for Nick and what he is going through is really wide. Lots of people want to see Nick feel better and succeed.

I love this quote by Alexandra Fuller in her autobiography of growing up in South Africa, *Don't Let's Go to the Dogs Tonight*: "This is not a full circle. It's life carrying on. It's the next breath we all take. It's the choice we make to get on with it." Fuller summarizes for me the peaceable way forward I am living as an autism mom right now. Nick is not recovered. He is healthier and happier than he has been since his regression, but he has a lot of hard work ahead. We are not in a perfect space as a family, but we are more than surviving, which is where we were just a few short years ago. We are moving forward with humor and grace and love.

SNAP OUT OF IT!!

"We believe Alexander has autism." My husband and I were sitting in a school supply closet with the school social worker as she said those words. She looked at us with so much pity; it was as if she'd just told us our child had died. Tears immediately fell from my eyes. My entire body went completely numb, and I couldn't breathe. It felt like a volcano had erupted inside of me. Every dream I had for my son vanished. I felt dead inside. Our son was only two and a half years old. It was September 22, 2003, at 8:22 AM; I remember it like it was yesterday. After hearing those words, my life has *never* been the same. To me, this date is as symbolic as September 11 is to our country.

I always felt like everyone around me was playing out "The Game of Life." You graduate high school, go to college, get married, have kids, live in a beautiful home, and have a beautiful life. I used to play this board game when I was younger. Now I realize that was more Fantasy Island than real life. Through my journey of having a child affected by autism, I have learned that it is all about keeping a positive attitude, never giving up, and realizing God chose me for a reason. It took me a while to get to where I am today, but I am so grateful that I am here. In the beginning, I was out of control and terrified of the unknown.

When our meeting ended, we walked out of the supply closet, and my husband said, "I will see you later," as he headed back to work. We didn't even look at each other. I don't think we could.

On my way out, I stopped and watched my son at play. He was lining up some ducks and then started playing with a gears game: just watching the gears with amazement, amused with the spinning vibrant colors. I felt a wave of deep love and knew I was going to burst into tears again, so I ran out.

I got into my SUV and thought, *What the hell just happened; how did I miss this?* I started thinking about Alexander's history. How did my son's pediatrician miss this? Why, after every well-baby checkup, did she tell me, "You have a healthy, happy baby"? Back in February, we went to the ENT to check our son's hearing, and he told us that Alexander's hearing was fine, that our son's condition was "normal," that he was just a "lazy talker." Alexander attended an educational day-care center. Why did they not catch this? I had expressed concern to them last May when I thought our son should be talking more, but they told me he was a boy, and this was normal.

As I drove home, I called my parents and some close friends. When I got home, I collapsed on my couch and cried for five hours. I remember our phones kept ringing and ringing, but I was too numb to answer. Finally, I had to stop crying and go pick up Alexander from day care. It was so hard to walk into that center; I now hated that place. I walked out clinging to my son. I held him so tightly it was as if I thought I could squeeze autism out of him. When we were driving home, I stared at him, wondering what his life was going to be like. Would he ever be able to talk to me?

My sister-in-law Kim called the next day to tell me she had talked to a professor named Gretchen from one of the major colleges who specialized in autism. Kim gave me Gretchen's phone number. (Kim is the queen of Google, and if anyone ever has a problem, Kim goes into research mode.) I thought it was possible that the social worker was wrong. I needed a professional's opinion, so I called Gretchen and scheduled an appointment with her in our home so she could meet Alexander.

It was a beautiful Saturday fall afternoon. My husband and my father left for the Michigan vs. Notre Dame football game, and my mom and I waited to meet Gretchen. I don't think my husband wanted to believe this was happening. When Gretchen arrived, she immediately went to my son and called his name. Alexander did not answer. She clapped her hands, and again he did not respond. She started blowing bubbles, and finally he responded, but only to the bubbles, not to her. She did a number of other things and talked with me for about two hours. Afterward, she confirmed, "Alexander has autism." I had missed every sign, but then again, I had no idea what autism was exactly. She gave us the name of a pediatric neurologist, Dr. Manico. The following Monday morning I called Dr. Manico's office to schedule an appointment.

Sitting in the neurologist's office, I thought to myself, *I can't believe we have to do this. This can't be happening to me.* When the doctor was ready to see us, we went into the exam room. He asked us some questions and said he really wasn't sure. *What?* So there was a glimmer of hope! He said we had to do an MRI and an EEG. Back then, I just did what the doctors told me to without question. I was afraid and did not even ask why. I don't think I wanted to know.

The MRI was not so bad except when I had to carry my screaming child into the room and hand him to the nurse. She told me not to worry and that they would be putting him under. The EEG, however, was the second worst day of my life. The doctor told me to schedule it during his nap time so Alexander would sleep through it. They couldn't sedate him for the EEG, as that would interfere with the test. Alexander fell asleep in my arms, and then the nurse put him in a papoose—in other words, a straightjacket. She had only put about half of the seventy-some electrodes on his head when Alexander woke up screaming and tried to move his little body. He was trapped. His entire body was wrapped so tightly it was like watching Houdini try to escape certain death, but this was my baby boy! I started crying as I tried to comfort him. We were torturing him. I screamed at the nurse to put a video on for him, something to distract him, but nothing worked. Alexander was in that papoose (straightjacket) for about twenty more minutes, screaming and crying, his face beet red. Finally, I couldn't take it anymore. I made them take him out. The nurse said it was fine, that they had completed the test. I furiously started undoing the fasteners. I sobbed as I held him and repeatedly told him I was so sorry and that Mommy would never let anything hurt him again.

After the MRI and the EEG came back normal, Dr. Manico concluded in his evaluation that Alexander was medically healthy. *Remember* this term: medically healthy. He referred us to Dr. Marsh, a licensed psychologist, for an evaluation of possible autism. I prayed and prayed, *Please, God, let it be something else, something that I can fix.*

My first impression of Dr. Marsh was that he reminded me of Gene Wilder in *Willy Wonka and the Chocolate Factory*. However, I was told he was one of the best. Dr. Marsh reviewed Alexander's history. He determined that my pregnancy was normal. Alexander was born through C-section and was a healthy baby but was now getting special education services for speech and occupational therapy once a week. His MRI and EEG were normal. Dr. Marsh observed Alexander but seemed to be more worried about him getting Cheerios on his twenty-year-old carpet than my son's behavior or medical condition. I remember thinking, *All doctors are useless*. I wanted them to give us some hope and tell us there was something we could do to help Alexander. Instead he told us, "Yes, he has autism." Again, my husband got in his car and went back to work. I got in my truck with Alexander and headed home.

I stared at Alexander (I found myself staring at him a lot) on the way home, and again I could not stop crying. When I pulled into our garage, I paused and thought, *Keep the truck running and close the garage*. I sat there for a few minutes, but it felt like hours. I looked in the back seat at my little boy's face and thought I can't kill my *baby*. My next thought was to kill myself, but then I thought I couldn't do that either because who would take care of Alexander? So many crazy things were running through my head. I then simply said a prayer and begged and pleaded with God to help me.

For the next three days, all I did was cry. I remember going to the park where I always took Alexander to play. It was pouring rain. I sat in my truck and cried hard for six hours. I was screaming at the top of my lungs, "Why my son? Why us?" My husband and I loved kids and could not wait to be parents. It was our dream. I yelled at God. I was in a fit of rage and completely out of control. I snapped!

I continued to cry all night while my husband tried to console me. The next morning he said to me, "You do whatever you have to do to help our son, and I will work 24/7 to pay for whatever his needs are. We are in this together." Then my husband showed me a sign he'd made and hung on our back door. It read, "We are going through this door today and we are going to beat the odds. Press this button for Super Positive

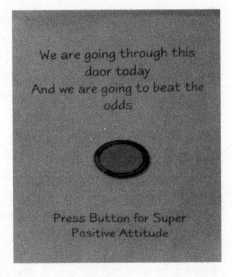

Attitude," and there was a big orange button. That sign is still on our back door today.

That afternoon, I laid on the couch and decided to read one of the three books about autism that my brother-in-law, Randy, bought for me. I picked one of Temple Grandin's books and could not put it down. I read the entire book and thought, *Wow! Alexander can get better.* That same day, Kim (Google Queen) called me to tell me about a doctor who did PLAY (also known as Floortime) therapy, which helped kids with autism. She emailed me the article and said the author would be speaking that following Saturday. Of course we went. There I met some other parents whose children had benefited from this type of therapy, so we signed up, and PLAY therapy began.

Next, I called one of the local hospitals to check into getting some type of speech therapy for Alexander. The woman I spoke to gave me the names and numbers of two women, Mary and Sara, who had "recovered" their children from autism. *Recovered?* The word took my breath away. I hung up and called Mary's number. She saved my life, and I will be forever grateful to her. She gave me the names and numbers for dozens of resources. She took me to the health food store and explained the gluten-free and casein-free diet. She invited me to join a support group, Everyday Miracles, for moms and dads of kids with autism. I no longer felt like I was alone. I also started to realize that there were many parents like me with children affected by autism. I still remember at my first meeting there was a little boy who asked his mom for some juice. The mom was excited and said to me, "He is just starting to talk." This gave me butterflies. Mary invited me to her home, and I met her son, who *used to have* autism. He was the cutest little boy. He talked to me, played with his toys, and even played the piano for me. As of that minute, I had a mission: I would recover my son.

It would take me forever to discuss in detail each therapy we did for our son, but here is the list: speech, occupational therapy, eating therapy, listening therapy, PLAY, RDI, and ABA (applied behavior analysis). We had, at one time, six different ABA therapists who came to our home for four hours twice a day. I remember the very first session. The therapist and my son sat facing each other, and she said, "Alexander, look at me," and grabbed his face and turned it toward hers. This went on for the entire session. I knew then that we had to teach Alexander to respond to his name.

One summer, I signed us up for a program in which the parents were taught how to do ABA therapy with their children. Every day for three months from nine to twelve, Alexander and I would drive forty minutes each way to therapy. I hated doing this; it was the summer from hell. However, it was probably one of the best things I did for him and for me. It taught me how to teach him. I remember watching Alexander during an occupational therapy session through the double-sided glass, sitting on a tire swing with headphones on, screaming and crying. I thought, *This is not my life; I am supposed to be at play dates and Gymboree class—anywhere but here.* It was heart wrenching to watch. In eating therapy, it took five months to get Alexander to eat a carrot, it took us a year to get him to eat foods other than the six he typically ate. We did a therapy called SMILE, during which he lay on a rotating bed in the pitch dark and stared at a light box that focused different colors on different parts of his brain. At the same time, he had a set of headphones that worked different parts of his brain. He had to do this for an hour, twice a day, for fourteen days straight. Finally, we had an "aha" moment. Alexander read the book, *The Very Hungry Caterpillar*—which he had not memorized. He read the book!

Remember the term "medically healthy"? In Alexander's case, this was the farthest thing from the truth. While doing all the different therapies I mentioned, we were also doing, and continue to do, biomedical treatments. We had to—and continue to—do urine, stool, and blood testing. We do homeopathy, HBOT (hyperbaric oxygen therapy), infrared sauna, neurofeedback, ZYTO (energy testing), and chelation.

We once saw a naturopathic doctor, who my mother was convinced was crazy. A friend had recommended him. He *was* a bit strange, but he might be able to help our son, so . . . yeah. My mom went with us. His office was in his house. As we drove up the long driveway, we noticed that the house was old, the windows were so dirty you couldn't see through them, and the yard was littered with statues and junk. My mom looked at me and said, "There is no way you are taking my grandson in there."

Just then, I saw a statue of the Holy Mother. My mom is a true, full-blown Catholic, so I said jokingly, "Oh look, Mom! The Holy Mother is here. She will protect us."

The entrance was in the back. When the doctor was ready for us, he walked us through a pitch-dark tunnel in his basement, which reminded me of Batman's Batcave. The whole time, my mom was poking me in the back, whispering, "Get us out of here. We are going to die."

We got to the exam room, home to thousands of tiny vials full of different elixirs. My mom continued to roll her eyes at me. We went back to this doctor a couple times, but after a while I realized that the visits were getting us nowhere.

Many doctors and therapists have told me autism is not a medical condition; children are born with it and it is neurological. Confused yet? I was. What happened to all the reports from the pediatrician that stated I had a healthy, happy baby? What happened to the little baby who played peek-a-boo with me or crawled up to his grandmother every time he wanted his bottle and said, "Ba bas?" Alexander slowly regressed into autism. Going back and looking at pictures from when he was born up until he was two years old clearly shows his decline. From birth, I had his picture taken every six months. His two-year-old picture is expressionless. I remember that day at the photographer's how he would not look at the camera or anyone else. He cried the entire time, but I thought he was just tired and cranky.

I later understood that Alexander had a vaccine reaction after his three-month well-baby visit. I remember being at the pediatrician's office crying and begging them not to give him four vaccines at once. The nurse reassured me saying, "It is safe. We do this all the time." Within ten hours, we were in the emergency room. My little baby's body was covered from head to toe, front and back, in a rash, and he was crying inconsolably. I called his pediatrician and said, "I was just in, and he had his vaccines" (thinking the vaccines were going to keep him healthy), and she said, "Oh, this is not from that." After two hours, the ER doctor told me he wasn't sure what it was and thought maybe eczema. It was not eczema; he had an allergic reaction to his vaccines. After this episode and more and more vaccines, he kept getting chronic ear infections. It seemed like every other month Alexander had an ear infection and sometimes a double ear infection. When I questioned his pediatrician about this, again she told me it was no big deal, very common in boys; it's "normal." Later, I found out this was a sign of a weakened immune system. Alexander had close to twenty vaccines before the age of two. I will not get stuck on the whole vaccine issue, but I will say that vaccines caused our son's autism, and they made my child medically sick.

Our son is now ten years old. He has not "recovered"—*yet*! For us, recovery means living independently, having a career he enjoys, and living a happy and healthy life—not society's so-called "Game of Life," but life on his terms. After all the trials and tribulations, Alexander has taught me more than I could ever have taught him. When I see how hard he works, it motivates me to work harder. I have learned about myself, and I think I have become a better person for it. I take nothing for granted and appreciate every little thing in life. It's funny how life works; if you want life to work, it does.

I no longer trust the majority of the mainstream medical community. I make all the decisions regarding my son's medical treatment. I have chosen doctors, homeopaths, and a nutritionist who understand autism and know how to treat it. I have learned so much from all the great moms and dads I have met over the years at numerous autism conferences, Yahoo! groups, and Facebook groups who are in this fight with me. I have found that parents of children with autism literally open their hearts to anyone and everyone who needs guidance and support while fighting for his or her own children. I believe that all the parents I have met through this journey are angels sent to me from God.

My husband and I always have had the attitude that even though our son is affected by autism, we are still going to continue to live our lives and not let our son's autism get in the way. We look at Alexander as our child and not a child with a disability. I don't panic anymore about every little thing. I remember always worrying: Will he be able to talk? Will he be able to ride a bike, swim, read, write? He now does all those things and much more. He learned them in his own time. Alexander is so loving. He adores his family. He has the best "Grammy" and "Papa" in the world. My parents have helped us on this journey and are in this fight with us. (Thank you, Mom and Dad. I love you.) Alexander loves going on vacations, especially with his cousins, Lily and Shayne. One of his favorite places to visit was Mount Rushmore. He now wants to go to the hot air balloon festival in Santa Fe, New Mexico. We are still working on many issues, such as social, sensory, and healing his sick body, but we will get there.

I know in my heart that someday Alexander will be healthy, and with God all things are possible. We love our son more than anything, and we cherish every moment with him and look forward to each day with him, waiting to see what wonderful things he will accomplish today. To every parent who has a child affected by autism, love your child where he or she is, and for all the positive things he or she does, but still keep fighting and *never give up!* *Recovery is possible, and it will happen.*

Bytes from the Count

Bob and Anita are good friends of mine. Bob is a bit of a rarity: He's one of the biomed dads who knows equally as much as the mom. And believe it or not, he's as equally gung ho as I am. I used to tell Bob how lucky he is that his wife is his biomed equal, as my wife knows nothing about it and can't stand more than three minutes of biomed talk. He tells me, no, I'm the lucky one because I get to decide everything. He says they usually quarrel over what biomed path to take.

They live in a different state, but I got to see them on a business trip once. I had lunch with Bob, and he told me, "I have something to confess. I've been cheating on Anita." I practically jumped out of my chair. I yelled, "Whoa, whoa! Don't lay this one on me! Whatever you're doing, I don't want to know!!" Bob laughed and said, "No, no! It's not what you think!" Apparently, they had been disagreeing over the dosage of a prescription supplement to give to their ASD son. Anita had instructed him to give a quarter of a capsule daily. He instead gave half a capsule and didn't tell her. Their son had been showing gains since he switched the dose, and Anita had been trying to attribute that to some other things since she didn't know. I said that in my humble opinion, they should give the whole capsule.

Bob called me a couple of weeks later. He said they bickered over some biomed things. Anita wanted to stop the supplement and try something else. He didn't want to stop. So, she hid the supplement so he couldn't give it anymore! He asked me to mail him a bottle on the down low to his work address so he can keep giving it. Great. Now I'm a drug dealer and a home wrecker.

Mamacita's Unexpected Gift

Have you ever dreamed of what your future was going to be like? Did you have a picture in your mind of exactly what you hoped? Did those dreams come to fruition just as you thought? Isn't it very rare that what you picture in your mind actually happens?

As the parent of a special-needs child, I could not predict that my child would have the difficulties he does now. For children who were born with delays, some prenatal testing may have been an indicator that issues would arise. Those parents might have had time to acknowledge that life would be completely different than they had planned. Maybe something could have predicted my child's delays, but doctors said that the baby growing in my womb looked fine. I had some experience with pregnancy and what to expect, because I had just had a little girl the year prior. I gained more weight with my second pregnancy, but scans showed a perfect baby in utero. My baby. My first boy. I was looking forward to bringing a newborn home again.

My little family was growing, just as I had hoped. I had just two more months to wait out the uncomfortable weight gain, and then Ronan arrived. He was born four weeks early but was healthy and had stellar Apgar scores. Indicators, and the reality of how drastically his health and my parenting would change, were never on my radar. Incredible excitement was the only thing I knew and felt as I held my brand new baby on his first day of life.

After bringing Ronan home from the hospital, we made it through his first month with chronic jaundice and a heart murmur scare. Ronan slept a lot those first few weeks, for which I was grateful. The jaundice slowly went away, and Ronan's heart checked out just fine. He started to grow as all good babies do and took lots of naps. Sleep for me was nonexistent. My almost two-year-old daughter, Fiona, had a toddler energy level and didn't understand how incredibly tired Mommy was. I looked like I hadn't slept in weeks (because I hadn't) when my seventy-three-year-old neighbor, a retired New York City policeman and fireman, reminded me one day when he came to visit, "Cathy, he's a beautiful baby. You're doing a great job with the two kids. Remember that these early weeks will get better. The first ninety days are tough, but you can't give the kid back. Just keep at it, and it'll get better. You can do it." I loved his fatherly advice and reminded myself daily that I could be strong enough to push through the initial stages of sleeplessness I was going through with a newborn and an active toddler.

Tending to two small children was a daunting task, but with Fiona's growing skills and helpful demeanor, I was lucky to have her around. My daughter's development was perfect. She'd gotten one ear infection at nine months of age and that was it as far as major sicknesses went. I had a very "textbook" example in my daughter's health—Fiona was normal in every stretch of the imagination. Her milestones were always met with ease and timeliness according to what the doctor and his charts expected at her well-baby checkups. The parenting website I used to track Fiona's development sent weekly messages about what I should see with her health and growth. It was like getting little high fives in my email inbox: Yes! She did it again . . . rolled over, sat up, pincer grasped, babbled.

Like clockwork, Fiona turned into a precocious toddler who was even teaching herself how to read at the age of three. Because I'd only just left the classroom after ten years of teaching when Fiona was born, I wasn't ready to turn my teaching brain off after she arrived. Naturally, I decorated and organized Fiona's playroom shelves with educational activities. I had a mini-me in the making who loved letters, books, writing, and reading. Fiona was happy and content with her toys and activities while pushing herself to try to do more. The little girl mothering skills Fiona naturally had were also a joy to see. She was always kind and considerate to Ronan, whom she affectionately called "Baby."

Baby grew from a four-week premature tiny little thing into a fat and happy baby. Ronan's big brown eyes soaked in everything he saw. The smile Ronan flashed made everyone melt. He was such a chunky chunk with dark, all boy, and beautiful features. I remember a conversation I had with my mom when Ronan was around two months old: "Mom, I know boys aren't supposed to be called beautiful, but Ronan is just that. He's gorgeous! I can't help but stare at him sometimes." With each passing day, I looked forward to what else Ronan would bring to my life. Fiona continued to be a doting big sister and loved being Mommy's special helper. My heart was full. I felt like I was at the top of the world as a young mother.

Having witnessed Fiona's recent milestone accomplishments and knowing what she was capable of doing as a typical baby was both a positive and a negative experience. Ronan gave me some scares early in life that didn't coincide with how I recalled Fiona developing. His first few months seemed uneventful as I was living through them, but later I had some thoughts that didn't sit well with me. "Huh, I don't remember that reaction happening to Fiona" when Ronan got some of his vaccines. I also thought, "He seems to be a tiny bit slower to do that same skill (like sitting up and rolling over) compared to big sister." I didn't want to dwell on those very subtle thoughts though. No one else shared my worry either as people told me, "Ronan is a boy; he'll catch up." Or, "He was premature. Give him some time." So, I gave him time and kept the nagging thoughts to myself.

I loved being a mommy to two little people. I kept busy or distracted from the concern I was desperately trying not to think about as Ronan went from a beautiful baby boy to his troubled toddler days. Other than that, life was mostly easy. We were living it happily, and I liked it.

Then, those pesky thoughts about Ronan's development started to invade again. The nagging and subsequent questioning of something not being entirely right with him became an everyday struggle. I knew what "typical" was supposed to look like. I knew that normal development shouldn't be an effort to accomplish. That's when I started to draw upon my memory of notes I took in my early childhood and education classes from college. I was constantly tested or asked to expand on typically developing skills most children experienced when I wrote my papers or presentations. I wanted to find those papers and study them again. I wanted to rewind back to those seminars I attended. I had observed countless hours of normal play from birth through preschool. I knew that what I was seeing in my son didn't fit the textbooks or the hands-on student teaching I experienced. Knowing what Ronan should be doing as a growing baby scared me because the reality of what he wasn't doing was not the "typical" I knew.

I had boxed up and stored all my college books, never expecting to use them so quickly after "retiring" from teaching. Fiona was born two months after my last teaching job ended. I longed to stay home with my baby and any more children I might end up having. I ended up finding the textbooks in the attic during the kids' naptime. I sat and thumbed through the early childhood texts first and marked places I wanted to go back to read. I felt silly going back to the books at one point because I thought, *What kind of mother studies her own child?!* But I knew that Ronan's next well-baby checkup was around the corner. I was thinking about asking our pediatrician if I had a reason to be concerned with the lack of development I thought I was seeing. I needed to prepare myself for whatever our doctor might say, so I kept on reading.

When I looked at Ronan through the eyes of a researcher instead of his mother, I could see clearly that he was not navigating the environment. I could see the slower signs of cognitive growth when compared to his big sister. The few textbooks I still had reminded me what "normal" should look like. I started taking mental notes of what should have happened and what was happening instead. I was determined to retrace my steps and Ronan's growth to find out how and exactly when Ronan fell off the developmental track. I wasn't ready to fully admit that Ronan had a big problem, nor did I believe he had any specific issue or disease yet. I did what most researchers do when they're faced with a dilemma: I went back to the beginning (Ronan's birth), documented what was known (looked through his medical records), asked hundreds of rhetorical questions (discovered this thing called a search engine named Google), created possible theories (diagnosed Ronan with every disease, syndrome, and medical death sentence known to man), and tried to prove them wrong (cried a lot).

When I had an hour to myself, I would race over to the community college library, where I could read or check out medical books. I checked every book out that I could carry. Topics ranged from allergies to psychotic episodes. Nothing I read was exactly what I thought Ronan was suffering. I knew it was something, but what? What was this thing making my son do what he was, or wasn't, doing? I was a mommy turned medical detective drawn to find out as much as I could about the human body. Once I scoured the medical section at my local college, I started to request books and material from the statewide community college library system. What I couldn't understand was that I knew whatever Ronan was suffering had to be medically related, but the textbooks were giving me no clear answers. Our doctor was also baffled and offered a "wait and see" approach. Other doctors I talked to were quick to offer drugs, more testing, and more drugs. Our family history brought up nothing significant. Long hours of reading, wondering, and dead-end medical appointments offered medical arrogance, frustration, and hundreds more questions than answers.

For years, Ronan and I made our way through the rounds of many specialists. Ronan was tested for several genetic and rare diseases. He went through hours of therapy and attended special schools. I read as much as I could to try to find an accurate diagnosis for Ronan, but I kept coming up short. We were living in a very small, rural town when Ronan tumbled off the path of typical childhood. Limited resources caused further aggravation and delays for Ronan's specific needs. He was slow to talk, very late to walk, ended up losing what little speech he had, and struggled to make cognitive, social, and emotional gains. No one in our town had a child like Ronan, which added to my struggle of understanding and accepting what my child was going through. I felt like everyone was staring at me and at him when he had an unexplained meltdown. I started to limit what events we went to and who we visited. I struggled greatly as Ronan aged and morphed from a fat, happy baby to a detached and hyperactive preschooler. I yearned for like-minded friends who could help me or at least let me cry out my frustration without being judged. I wanted to take my kids to the park or on play dates where Ronan wasn't stared at or reprimanded for going where he didn't understand he couldn't go. Ronan was getting older, and his behavior was becoming increasingly strange. I was beyond tired and getting scared about Ronan's slowed development. It was time for some serious changes.

My sister suggested I join an online message board after hearing about the lack of answers I was getting locally. I searched the Yahoo! groups, which were rising in popularity. I found several groups I could call "home" that were parent-based yet medically minded. Finally! I was having conversations with people who knew exactly what Ronan was doing. They even suggested how to get diagnosis information from professionals, what tests to request, and how to treat the symptoms that I was seeing. Nameless people I could only recognize from a screen name from the other side of a computer became my friends, my confidants, and my lifeline.

I can't say I fully accepted the struggles Ronan had even with the support of my newfound friends, but I know that the bond created by the parents on those message boards got me through some of the darkest hours I have ever experienced as a parent. The closer I got to securing an exact diagnosis for Ronan, the more confident I became in my new role as advocate for Ronan. Every step closer to knowing what it was Ronan had, and learning every reason why he did what he did, was still hard to swallow. But it was more bearable to make decisions for Ronan. Having a link to other parents,

some who were years ahead of me in finding out their child's diagnosis, gave me strength to deal with the human beings standing next
to me who could see that Ronan needed a ton of help but later
refused to listen or act on my concerns.

None of this was easy. I wanted to run away from the constant
struggles I was facing—professionals who could have diagnosed
Ronan in those early years of questioning refused to help. People
who were supposed to teach him didn't; and worse than that, they
abused his right to an education. Ronan missed out on some hopeful treatment and on the chance to get closer to typical because of
the pride and greed other people put in front of his needs. I could
find helpful private programs for Ronan, but his therapy and education cost more than we could afford.

Our family had grown again, and my level of patience and
energy were completely zapped. My bubble of simple, happy parenting threatened to burst the longer I lingered on the message
boards, reading everyone's stories. Hearing their struggles and
knowing the connections many of us were making to environmental triggers that lead to our children's poor health depressed me.
Most of my free time, in between chasing Ronan to do what he
was supposed to do while taking care of my other children, was
spent on the Internet. I looked up every single word I read or heard
that might bring me closer to a diagnosis for Ronan. It wasn't just
the diagnosis I wanted. I knew that if I could name this thing that
Ronan had, I could ask for effective treatment for him.

To add to the stress, I didn't know how to slow down because
of how quickly I thought about Ronan. Ronan, his behaviors, his
delays, my husband's job and traveling demands, my other children and their busy lives—all swirled round and round in my mind.
I constantly craved to get online to try to figure out whatever it was
that Ronan had. But my life was so full of other things. I was desperate to find treatment to fix whatever I could to make Ronan's
life easier for him, thinking that if I can do that, the rest of life
would settled down just a little bit for me.

I spent more time on the message boards and made more
hypotheses about Ronan. I started to neglect household chores.

I even let the TV and DVDs "babysit" my typical kids so I could steal a few moments and hide out longer on the computer. Nothing I looked up confirmed every symptom Ronan suffered. He started to get worse with each sickness as he aged—bouts of a typical cold lasted longer and hit him harder than everyone else in the house. When Ronan lay so ill in the emergency room several visits in a row, I promised I would continue to fight for him as well as find a proper diagnosis.

Therapies, as well as some of Ronan's helpers, were helpful, but the assistance never seemed enough. Ronan was a complicated kid who fit into one diagnosis one day and another one a different day. The inconsistency was so great that I felt forced to continue to explore a medical explanation. I knew I needed to find doctors who were able to run lab tests of all kinds: genetic, metabolic, brain, gut, ears, eyes, heart, urine, feces, hair, blood. You name it and Ronan gave it or was tested for it. His sensory issues prohibited some testing opportunities and certain therapies. I hated how his sensory defensiveness intruded the everyday living Ronan had to do. I hated it even more when a potential test or evaluation that could lead to a diagnosis was interrupted or made impossible by Ronan's severe issues. He'd hit all manner of roadblocks, which could make a giant step forward turn into a tumble backward beyond the original starting point. It made any progress insignificant.

I'd walked into so many exam rooms from Ronan's early toddler days through his early school-age years. I'd always keep my hopes thinking that the next lab-coated individual would be "the one" to give me helpful answers. Some doctors were very well educated, but they weren't very focused on Ronan. One group of specialists only wanted to push their high-dose prescription on us after I'd asked—no, begged—"Please! Aren't there vitamins or supplements or a special diet?" Those seizure doctors from a very large university hospital said no and only offered us drugs that we later learned could have caused a serious reaction. Ronan should never have been given such a high dose of the drug, nor should he have been on it for the duration he took it.

I lost a lot of faith, trust, and hope for much of the medical field as I wandered from one clinic to the next. Doctors and nurses gave me the once over if I mentioned we were delaying vaccines. They came very close to accusing me of jeopardizing the rest of the human population by not vaccinating Ronan. How dare I?! If they'd only stop and really look at Ronan's medical history and how it tied into his medical mysteries, they would have understood my logic and respected that what I was saying was exactly what some of their peers were publishing.

One particular doctor brought more doom, gloom, and disrespect than anything else. He was the most disheveled, pompous, unprofessional doctor we dealt with to date. To add insult to injury, the guy was incredibly late to a very nerve-wracking appointment. We felt forced to stay through it because he was the doctor who could order several panels of tests that might very well give us a diagnosis for Ronan. The encounter was early on in Ronan's medical journey, when I could barely pronounce some of the technical words and scientific terms I was reading. A fellow message-board parent read a post I wrote on the board the day before this big appointment. I'd described the clinic Ronan was going to and asked for advice on what I should ask of the doctor. Several people chimed in with suggestions, and others sent good-luck messages. A parent wrote back and said what I described sounded a lot like mitochondrial disease. I had skimmed a few articles that mentioned the condition so I could be more familiar it. The more I read, the more I thought that mito made a lot of sense to pursue. I added mito disease to my very long list of questions and concerns to bring to the new doc.

So, as my husband and I nervously waited for what we hoped would be the day we got some big questions answered, the doctor, who was also arrogant, tardy, and sloppy, fumbled his way into the exam room that Ronan was trying hard to stay in. This day also included other tests and exams, and Ronan was already agitated with the amount of waiting he'd had to do. It was getting difficult to keep Ronan entertained and away from the exam room door.

We thought we had waited far longer than we should have when all of a sudden the door flew open. In walked a doctor with papers falling out of his overstuffed briefcase. He barely said hello before making pathetic excuses for why he was late (which was because "I knew you would be here no matter how late I was because you had an appointment before mine and another one sometime after mine"). He proceeded to ignore Ronan, who was ready to claw his way out of the tiny room, while making sure to tell us how important and full of himself he was.

The doctor started off describing some reports from Ronan's files and then shot off some names of tests he wanted to run on Ronan. I nodded my head and tried to remember the description of the labs as well as the diseases they might help us discover. I calmed myself down since some of the genetic issues he listed sounded eerily familiar. Then he asked if my husband or I had questions before asking us to agree to the blood work he wanted done. I sat up and asked if Ronan could have mitochondrial disease, because his symptoms fit the description I had reread the night before, right before I turned the Internet off. The doctor looked insulted as I finished my question. He shot back a verbal slap across my face, and he glared. Never in my wildest dreams did I expect anything I might say would insult a doctor's medical intelligence, but apparently I did. It was a simple question that had every bit of logic attached to it. My husband was floored that this doctor would react so negatively to a legitimate concern we both held. The doctor said no to the testing, and he said it emphatically.

Since the doctor wouldn't allow us to go forward with the mitochondrial disease testing, my husband picked up Ronan and left the appointment. I was determined to stay in my seat. I waited until the doctor fully explained why he refused to sign off on a simple lab that could potentially end all of the searching I was doing. He babbled about how expensive the test was and how inconvenient it would be to get the blood work to the lab that did that testing. He made so many excuses and said he wouldn't take part in it. I grilled him further until we were at a standstill. The doctor wouldn't budge. All I could do was leave that tiny exam room full of tension. Anger filled my being. I just couldn't understand why someone wouldn't listen. It wasn't like he was going to have to pay the bill for the lab. And he wasn't going to be the one to take care of a potentially chronically ill child: I was! It took three more years and many more medical professional discussions before I finally got someone to order the mito lab test. When the results came back, they confirmed that yes, my mommy gut was right: Ronan had a mitochondrial disease.

Through all of my reading, questioning, and observing, I couldn't help but think that Ronan was my own personal science experiment. I put him under so many microscopes, wondering why he suffered from problems my other children breezed through. I questioned why his health deteriorated so quickly after exposure to a viral infection. I feared that his illnesses were becoming too frequent and stacking one on top of the other. I always went back to the Internet to try to connect the information I had on my son, his development, and his continued struggles with anything that made sense. I read hundreds of medical links and journals, and searched websites that shared anecdotal input from other parents about their all-too-familiar stories of their children.

In the meantime, I felt like I was dealing on the black market when I began biomedical treatment for the gastrointestinal problems that plagued Ronan. From other parents' stories I'd heard that if you address the gut issues, cognitive gains could follow. Herbal remedies, homeopathy drops, special diets, and lots of poop being monitored became a way of life. Ronan had constant constipation that I couldn't get to budge. Ronan would start to limit what he ate when his tummy was bloated. He'd go up to five days without pooping, despite my efforts with natural remedies to encourage motility. Regular doctors only wanted to see Ronan on Miralax, but it was ineffective and actually caused worse problems. Taking matters into my own hands again, Ronan started the gluten-free, casein-free diet, and I further investigated digestive enzymes.

I started the dietary intervention when he was still unable to walk. Ronan was two and a half and had been using a walker for several months. The kid would zoom all over the hallways, through the aisles in stores, and everywhere we'd go. It was a temporary fix to a much greater neurological issue, but the walker gave Ronan the get-up-and-go his own body was unable to provide. Once I introduced digestive enzymes, we hit the jackpot with his very delayed gross motor skills. Three days after Ronan started taking the enzymes, he walked. He walked right into our church on a Sunday morning and didn't stop. The youth group had been praying for Ronan for several weeks, so we made our way over the parish hall and showed those young teens that prayers can indeed be answered.

Ronan continues to be a special-needs child. He has an unknown mitochondrial disease that looks like autism but isn't exactly autism. Some days he is on task making connections cognitively, emotionally, and physically. He walks like a regular kid. He plays with toys like they are meant to be played with. But on other days Ronan struggles to walk and tires easily. He doesn't respond as quickly and can also look as if he's losing a skill he had already gained. The progressive nature of the mito issues can cause great energy issues. It takes more coordination, stamina, and will power for Ronan to get from one place to the next. On those days, Ronan has a harder time eating, walking, working, and even relaxing. I'm sure he goes through pain, but Ronan has yet to regain his speech, so he can't say if something hurts or not. I still observe and analyze his every moment because Ronan can't tell me, "Hey, Mom, today sort of stinks. I need an extra few minutes, okay?"

Some days I feel like I am on an unending roller coaster of "what ifs" that still don't make sense. But Ronan has taught me more than I ever expected to learn as a parent. Even though I really only thought I'd be a mommy for this child, Ronan turned me into someone stronger and braver. I couldn't do what I need to without his peace and determination. I get a chance to do things I never knew existed. Not everything is easy, but I get to hope through every single one of Ronan's days: good days that wipe away sorrow and sadness, and bad days that bring me back to my knees praying for another opportunity to help my child.

I may never be able to understand or find solid answers for all of my questions about Ronan. I wonder if it would truly help me to know every single answer. Those answers, and the feelings I'd get from knowing them, might not make Ronan completely better. They're not a guarantee that he'd be stronger or easier to care for. It might make me feel empowered to have the medical or diagnostic explanation for the "if this, then that" reasoning. But, I want to also enjoy the life Ronan does have in that moment. Some days are so hard to push through, so I draw on the strength it takes to be able to go forward even one tiny step. Ronan's given me dreams, friends, and an attitude that no one else could ever provide. He's not what I expected as I carried him through pregnancy. He's far different than what I ever imagined. Even through the delays that slow him down today, Ronan's life gives me a steady beat that keeps me living, learning, and hoping for healing.

Bytes from the Count

I was talking to my DAN! doc. We talked about raising the secretory IGA because my son's is low. He asked if I'd like to try oral IG as opposed to IVIG. Oral is $200 a month as opposed to $2,000 for IV. It's not absorbed very well but is worth a try. It's once a week for a total of four doses in a month. I told him I'd try, and I left. Two days later a package arrives from the compounding pharmacy. I'm excited to try it. I open it up, and there are four syringes with huge honking needles on them and four vaccine-type bottles. The bottles say immunoglobulin for intramuscular use only—not to be taken orally. I think, *Oh crap, he must've decided to give me this instead*, and I think, *Well, let's go for it.* I extract the fluid. My son is screaming because he's about to get a shot. My wife is screaming because I'm giving the shot. I jabbed his butt and only partially put the needle in. I pushed very slowly because there was a lot of fluid, and it created a big bubble on his butt at first, but it disappeared. After it was done, I was thinking, "Man, that was not pleasant to give!"

The next morning, I'm drinking coffee and I look down on the counter . . . there's the bag with the rest of syringes. I see the pharmacy label says:

Patient: Johnny Doe

Directions: Extract fluid with syringe, squirt in mouth !@#!#@! Holy crap!

I called my doctor, and he immediately called the pharmacy to chew them out about the labeling on the bottles. He said no harm was done. It still gets absorbed, just a little differently!

I told one of my friends this story. He admits to me that when he first got transdermal glutathione . . . it came in syringe. So he was squirting it in his son's mouth for a couple days! Guess he missed the part about "transdermal."

HAVING MY CUPCAKE AND EATING IT TOO

A swell of emotion filled my chest. I birthed my first baby on a cold and wet March afternoon, and he was perfect. The first-born grandson on both sides of the family . . . what joy! We were all so excited to finally meet the little guy. The nurses all started referring to him as "The King of *Everything*," and he really was. He was certainly *my* everything—something I would prove time and again while advocating for my son. I was so happy to be a new mom, so desperate to bond with my son and be the best parent. I certainly expected bumps in the road; however, I did not expect a mountain to rise up in front of us.

I was told to try nursing Pooka, but he really fussed and struggled to latch on. "Don't worry," said the nurse. We're all new at this, and you both need a little practice." I was exhausted from eight hours of labor but kept trying to nurse the boy. He was so hungry and impatient that I laughed a little and told him, "Relax, food is coming." While I did manage to nurse him, he still fussed. My milk had not come in yet, and the colostrum was proving insufficient to the point that Pooka seemed to be starving. The nurse took him to the nursery to give me time to eat and rest. That night they kept bringing the baby back to me to nurse, but he couldn't really latch on, so he cried and cried. The staff finally convinced me to give up nursing and put him on formula. It was easier for him to eat from the bottle, so I agreed, and the lactation nurses and pediatrician felt that the problem was resolved. Yet I wondered what was so different or difficult about taking the breast. Everyone assured me it was fine and these things were normal.

At seven weeks of age, our baby slept through the night for the first time! That was the exact moment when he began crying, no . . . *screaming* throughout the day. From what seemed like the moment he woke up to the moment he fell asleep at night, Pooka would scream and scream and scream. I began to panic and asked other moms and the pediatrician questions. The crying was coupled with projectile vomiting and severe diarrhea. Pooka would also clench himself so tightly that he could not nap. I was beginning to lose my mind. There was something wrong with my baby, and no one seemed to care. My husband worked and attended graduate school in the evenings, so I had limited help. I started calling him home at lunch so he could pace around the house and try to get our child to sleep so I could have at least five minutes of peace. That pacing often put the little Pooka to sleep long enough for my husband to walk out the door to go back to work. Some days the crying was so bad it felt as though my skin was crawling with ants that kept biting and making me itch. I could have easily scratched off my skin and would have never known.

When I insisted our pediatrician look into the constant screaming, projectile vomiting, and chronic diarrhea after months of pleading, he finally recommend changing our formula from dairy to soy. Soy only made things worse. Pooka developed eczema, and he began to stink. A predigested formula was next, and it seemed to help with the gut pain enough so that he wouldn't scream *all* day, but the terrible diarrhea didn't go away. During this time, he never wanted to be held. I could hold my baby only so long as it took to feed him, and then I had to set him down again. The swing was the only thing that would comfort him. I had this beautiful baby boy whom I cherished with all my being, and I couldn't figure out what was wrong or comfort him in any way.

Was parenting really that difficult, or did I just have no clue? I repeatedly asked the doctor about the chronic diarrhea, and he told me that it was normal for some kids, especially babies. I asked about allergies and was told that he was too young. When I asked why our son didn't like to be held, he looked me square in the eye and suggested that I relax and have a glass of wine with lunch: "You'll feel better about you and your baby." I was on the hunt for a new doctor at this point but struggled to find one who would take me seriously.

We were well known at the local pediatricians' offices and at the ER. Little Pooka kept developing severe ear infections that were difficult to treat. A steady diet of antibiotics made his diarrhea worse. The poor boy's rear was so raw and miserable. He didn't want to be held but hated to be put down. I was really losing my mind and had no idea what to do. My attention was distracted from Pooka's problems for a little bit while we sold our house and were waiting for our new one to be finished. In the meantime, we moved to the city with my mom. I hoped to get a little help with Pooka, and I also hoped that I might get more help trying to figure out what was wrong.

As his first birthday drew nearer, I found myself concerned about his speech. He neither babbled nor talked. "He's a boy . . . All boys are late talkers. We have late talkers in the family, and they all turned out fine. Quit worrying so much," was what everyone told me. I wasn't convinced. There were clearly troubles in the beginning, but no one listened. People blamed me: I was the overly paranoid new mom who fussed over everything. Later, we learned that I wasn't paranoid and overly fussy. I was a mother in tune with her baby—an ability I lost when he later regressed and turned inward.

After Pooka was born, we realized we had to find a home with a yard, so we put our townhome on the market. We opted to build a house further out in the suburbs and enjoyed the extra help from my mom during the process. It was nice to have that help, and I enjoyed walking the neighborhood with him and doing our daily stroll to the grocery store for our dinner ingredients. Except for the troublesome ear infections, things seemed a bit easier.

We had a routine doctor's appointment, and Pooka was due for shots. Since we were nearing the end of our antibiotic and his ears were looking better, the pediatrician suggested we go ahead with the shots at this appointment to save us a trip. I wondered if this was a good thing to do while he was on antibiotics, but the doctor assured us Pooka would be fine. He was wrong.

By the time we were halfway back to Chicago, Pooka started this screeching sort of cry and developed a fever. I had no idea at this point that I should be very concerned—if not afraid—of what was happening to my baby. That was the last day he laughed and looked at us. That was the day my precious boy disappeared and was replaced by a stranger. I felt him drifting further away from me and didn't know what to do. No one else around me seemed to notice. If I confided in people, they'd roll their eyes and tell me things were fine. How were they going to react when I told them that I thought Pooka's soul was no longer in that chubby little toddler body? I tried my best to ignore what I was seeing, or rather what I was *not* seeing, and focused on the house.

The closer it got to moving day, the more odd behaviors Pooka exhibited. He started walking on his toes, flapping his hands, shaking his head from side to side, looking at things out of the corner of his eyes, spinning nonstop . . . and not talking. Every alarm was going off in my body. My heart would race, pressure would build in my head, and my body would tingle. Pooka also seemed to have gone deaf. He wouldn't respond to his name when called. To my heartache, he wouldn't turn to look at us or try to locate a loud noise. We got an appointment at Children's Memorial Hospital in Chicago to have his hearing tested. It was normal. We had them look at the toe walking, and they blamed it on the walker I used. No suggestions were made to correct the toe walking; it was assumed that Pooka would grow out of it.

After we moved into our new home, I was watching the *Today* show. It was a special on autism. My world crumbled. Pooka had autism. I knew right then. I called my mom upset and crying. She assured me I was wrong. There was no way it was autism. He was too smart and loved hugs (from her . . . not me). There was no way he had autism. My best friend also assured me that there was no possible way and to not get myself so upset. I wanted to believe they were right, but I knew deep in the pit of my stomach that they were wrong.

We began Early Intervention to get started with speech therapy and occupational therapy. Sadly, I didn't see any improvements and instead saw Pooka become more rigid from the tasks they taught him. I resented these therapists for making our son more distant than he already was. Their job was to turn that around, not make it worse. I began to look for private therapists and made an appointment to get a diagnosis.

After seeing us for only about fifteen minutes, the doctor told us Pooka was too young to diagnose at the age of two years and two weeks. Perhaps they could diagnose him in a year. In the meantime, the doctor wanted us to look into autism and PDD-NOS. He also mentioned that although he could not diagnose Pooka, he did suggest preparing ourselves for our future. That future would include a son that might not talk, learn to use the toilet, or tie his shoes. My fear became reality. A professional also considered this thing that was happening to Pooka was autism. It wasn't just me. When I called and spoke to my mom, she was crushed, but she also remained rational: "Okay, so how do we fix this?" With that, the crusade began. I wanted my baby back. I wanted to be able to look him in the eye, to tell him I loved him, and to know that he understood what I was saying to him. I wanted to hold my child and squeeze him, tickle him, and make up for all the time I missed.

While researching online, I kept coming across the gluten-free, casein-free (GFCF) diet and DAN! (Defeat Autism Now!) doctors. I showed some of the links to Ryan, my husband, and he was compelled to start the diet and call some of these DAN! doctors. We were put on a couple of waiting lists and scheduled an appointment with the Pfeiffer Treatment Center (PTC). Then we began researching the details of the diet.

I remembered working with a woman who did autism advocacy work, so I called and left a message letting her know we might have a child on the autism spectrum. She called back and told me her story. Her son had autism. They did the GFCF diet and saw a DAN! doctor (the same one at PTC), and she explained the progress they saw with him. I was convinced this was the road we needed to take, and so it began.

A couple of days after taking away dairy products, Pooka looked sick. He looked so pale, but wait . . . he was looking at me! He looked straight at me and smiled! I didn't understand. Why did he look so sick but look so good at the same time? He had been off dairy for two days. Could that explain the sudden gain of eye contact? But why was he so pale? I didn't care—he was in a great mood and was looking at me! I swooped him up and gave him a hug while he battled against me to get down. I set him down, expecting him to run off like he always did, but he just stood there. He looked up at me and smiled. He flapped a little and looked like he wanted to be picked up. My heart was ready to explode! I picked Pooka up, but he wanted down pretty quickly. So, I set him down again, but he didn't run off. He kept looking at me, and then he giggled. This boy had the most infectious giggle you'd ever heard (*everybody* described it with those exact words). I started to giggle, too, and then I sobbed. Off he went to play by himself somewhere in the house. I went to clean up my face in the bathroom, and when I walked out, the family photos on the wall caught my eye. The little boy in the pictures wasn't healthy. All the photos on the wall showed a bloated, chubby baby with flame-red cheeks and ears and dark circles under his eyes. I immediately decided we were pulling all gluten out of the house and grabbed the trash can.

A few days later, after removing gluten from the diet, I turned the corner to walk into the kitchen and saw the pantry door open. As I approached the door ready to close it, I found Pooka nearing the *top shelf*, grabbing at the box of Cheerios. It fell to the floor, and he dove off after it. My heart raced trying to figure out what was going on. I was wrestling him on the ground, away from the gluten-filled cereal, all the while wondering who let the badger in the house. Pooka was clawing at me to keep me away while he did his best to shovel what cereal he could get into his mouth. He threw tantrums the rest of the day, and his ears and face were back to being red. I was shocked to see how he was reacting. I got on one of the many autism-related Yahoo! groups I had joined and found out Pooka was detoxing the gluten and going through some major opioid withdrawal. Great, now my kid was a little junkie! I decided it would be wise to keep this bit of information out of the ears of our family. They all would have probably thought we'd seriously lost our minds with all this alternative diet and holistic mumbo jumbo.

The new diet did wonders, but it also made life difficult. No matter where we went, we had to drag a cooler full of food. Some people understood and tried to be accommodating, whereas others either ignored us and the fact that our son couldn't eat certain foods or were annoyed by it. We did learn a great deal about our friends and families through it all. We tried really hard not to make anyone feel obligated to change meal plans or recipes. Some people just couldn't understand the diet and Pooka's new needs, so we had to limit our time spent with those people and even less with the people who didn't believe us. They were the ones who felt the need to feed him things they knew he couldn't have.

We liked our DAN! doctor and were learning so much about the American diet, the chemicals in our food, clothing, actually in everything, as well as the vaccine schedule. We were horrified. We did our best to green our lives and started to eat more organic food. However, Pooka's skin would still flare up with eczema from time to time. A particularly bad case merited yet another trip to the doctor, and this time I demanded more specific answers. The doctor ordered a bunch of tests—everything from urine and stool to blood work and allergy testing. He assured us we'd get to the bottom of it.

A large manila envelope arrived containing our lab results. It was thicker than a telephone book. I was a bit excited to open the package, and I spread it all out on the floor in the family room so I could take a good look at everything at once. That's when I noticed the allergy testing. Wait . . . did that say he was *severely allergic to milk*? I think my heart stopped beating for about five minutes. I had a lump in my throat, and I felt sick. No wonder he was such a miserable little boy. I was basically poisoning him! He was a 5+ on the report, which I understood to mean anaphylaxis.

Another major offender was soy, which explained the eczema. *Everything* had soy in it. I was going to have to get rid of a lot of food again. The idea of it all exhausted me. Never mind the fact that there were many more offending foods on the list that I was regularly feeding to our son.

At the same time, we were seeing some pretty terrible behaviors. Pooka would hit himself and bounce his head off walls, the couch—you name it. He would even run a full-on sprint from one end of the house to the other and throw himself into the wall. This is how he spent many days. According to the labs, the clostridia count was high in the stool test. We used supplements to get rid of it only to then find out that he would get an intestinal yeast overgrowth. When his yeast was high, Pooka would spin all day, shake his head, and flap more. When the clostridia went up, he would get aggressive and start trashing the house—nothing like an extended ride on the gut bug teeter-totter! Some of these behaviors became learned behaviors, but we found a private OT who did an awesome job redirecting him and replacing the behaviors. We still had a long road, but Pooka was slowly getting better. *Very* slowly.

Pooka wasn't always a responder like some other kids I knew. Some kids had remarkable gains on the diet alone or with B12 shots, cod liver oil, enzymes, or vitamin D. We weren't ever really sure if we were seeing improvements on any of those things or not. A friend suggested I start using an online evaluation program that we could fill out before and after we tried something new. After doing that, we realized Pooka really was getting better but wasn't making those huge leaps like everyone else. Our DAN! doctor seemed to be running out of ideas, and we were getting discouraged. Around that time, we got a call from another DAN! doctor (we had forgotten that we had put ourselves on her waiting list over a year prior), who told us she had an opening. If this wasn't a sign from heaven, I wouldn't know what was!

In hindsight, both doctors were phenomenal. However, the second one didn't have any restrictions based on the clinic's research methodologies. So, we did see better results with her. She suggested we do some new genetic testing. Once the results were back, we saw that Pooka's body couldn't process sulfur products, which was upsetting because most of his supplements were sulfur based! The protocol the new doctor suggested was nearly the death of me. At one point, Pooka was taking minute amounts of nearly thirty supplements every day. Would I do it again? Yeah, probably. Why? Because my son got better! This is when he finally stopped having chronic diarrhea. Pooka was four years old. Four years of chronic diarrhea is insane.

People often ask if we had a "wow" moment. If I had to pick a moment, besides the realization that the diet worked wonders, I'd have to say it was milk thistle. After a suggestion that we do some light liver support, I decided to add it in. About two or three days in, I was working at my desk and was deep in thought. I heard something that didn't register in my head. I turned and saw Pooka there holding a small plastic *dinosaur*. Then I heard that sound again. A sound I didn't recognize. My brain was very slowly turning, and it registered that Pooka's mouth had been moving when I heard the sound. That "sound" was Pooka saying, "Dinosaur?" His first word was dinosaur? Not only was he talking, he was actually asking me a question! I was stunned. He was so patient with me being so slow to respond to him that he asked me again, "Dinosaur?" "Yes, *yes*! It's a dinosaur! The dino says 'Rawwr.'" I went overboard with the "Rawwr," and he ran off. I was literally bouncing up and down in my seat.

Pooka still really struggled with speech therapy even though he was getting speech therapy at school and privately. Words came very slowly. We wound up with a dyspraxia/apraxia diagnosis for Pooka. It seemed like everything we did gave him very minute gains and frustrated us in the process. We were grateful to his first teacher though. She was a kind woman, and Pooka seemed to like her a great deal. She tried her best to accommodate our needs and the food allergies and restrictions. We certainly butted heads on a number of occasions (much more than we'd like to admit); however, we had a mutual respect for each other and understood that we were both doing what we knew best for Pooka. We didn't necessarily have that experience with therapists and other teachers later with Pooka's schooling. Early on, we were lucky to have Mrs. Heath, and he grew very close to her. Pooka and I still struggled with our personal relationship, and he kept me at arm's length.

At an annual review meeting with our special-education cooperative, we were told that Pooka was ready to go into kindergarten. The team of educators said that they'd like to see him spend part of the day in the typically developing kindergarten classroom. We were elated! Everyone's hard work—his especially—had paid off. Little did we realize, it was the beginning of a downward spiral and a tumultuous relationship with our special education co-op.

Mrs. Benedict liked to make people think she was sweet, kind, and accepting, but this was only true if one didn't challenge her. The minute Pooka began to struggle with her classroom full of chaos, she removed Pooka and his aide from the room. We didn't realize how loud the classroom was and that it really bothered those sensitive ears. When Pooka's aide wasn't sensing his frustration, Pooka didn't have the words to tell anyone, so he began hitting his aide. That prompted the principal to call us into his office for a meeting. We knew that wasn't a good sign. We discovered things to be even worse when the principal threatened to have Pooka kicked out of school! That started our fight. That man threatened to kick a five-year-old out of school because his staff couldn't "control him." We politely asked what the antecedents were—a term he was unfamiliar with but should have known. At the end of our meeting, we had educated *him* on special education and the laws that govern it. The principal still gave us a stern warning that something needed to be done. He was right. We called the special-ed director and called an emergency IEP (individualized education plan) meeting.

A behavior plan was put into place, but Mrs. Benedict made it very clear that she no longer wanted our son in her class. She couldn't concentrate on her children who had the ability to learn. At that point, I was more than happy to take Pooka out of her class. We weren't sure that a negative environment like hers was a good idea. A new teacher, Miss Andrews was a delight! She had pretty, red, curly hair, and Pooka instantly fell in love. He really grew in her classroom. She knew how to challenge him and realized that he needed to be in an accelerated program. Pooka grew very close to her, and he worked very hard. I was happy with his academic growth, but we still weren't seeing much language. Labeling things and making simple requests were already established, but he only used about three words at a time. He was still very far behind his peers.

The following year proved to be worse in many different ways. Pooka's teacher, Mrs. Deville, was new to our district, and many of the former teachers left due to district budget cuts. The result, we later realized, was inferior teachers with little to no experience. We were optimistic going in, but we should have been very leery. Mrs. Deville struggled in the beginning of the year, and we later learned that she actually tried to quit after the first month of school. The co-op refused to let her out of her contract, and her attitude about it showed—she completely checked out. Pooka struggled even more. We were constantly having emergency meetings to figure things out. It was made clear to us that the majority of the staff had no clue how to handle kids with special needs. We forced the district staff to test him because we felt that some of his behaviors were due to boredom. When we saw the work Pooka was doing, we realized that he had been doing the same work for the past two years. No wonder the child was bored! Mrs. Deville flat out refused to change her teaching method and her curriculum, so another battle ensued. It was frustrating that we were the ones who had to educate the educators. They were grossly underqualified and lacked the will to do the right thing and educate themselves.

That was when the call came. "Come get Pooka. We can't handle him anymore." I was confused by the statement "We can't handle him anymore." What did that mean? I got to the school, and someone escorted me to a small room that was supposed to be an office. When we came around the corner, I saw three people peering in through a small window. I was really confused and didn't know what to expect. I approached the window and was able to get a view into the room only after Pooka's aide made a tally mark on a clipboard. What I saw terrified me more than anything in all my life. Pooka was running as fast as he could all around that room, throwing himself head first into the cinderblock walls, then he'd fall on the floor and claw at himself. I pushed everyone else away and opened the door. The minute he heard the knob turn, Pooka looked at the door, saw it was me, and literally flew toward me to attach himself to me. He was screaming like someone was skinning him alive. When I looked at his face, I went cold—he looked demonic, like a tortured soul sent to hell. His pupils were dilated so wide that you couldn't see any of the crystalline blue. He actually reminded me of Bruce, the shark from *Finding Nemo*, who'd turn diabolic at the scent of blood. Pooka was trembling violently and nearly in convulsions.

I started yelling, "What the hell is going on here? What did you do?" No one had an answer. They just stood and stared at me. I took him home as fast as I could. Pooka sobbed for the rest of the night, and I just held him. I promised my son I was going to do whatever I could to take the pain away and to make him happy. My anger and sadness felt like a knife plunged and twisted into my heart. I was terrified to think of what could have happened to make him react the way he did. Was he being abused? Was there some other underlying condition we were not aware of? What could it be?

I refused to send Pooka to school until the district answered my questions. We demanded an outside evaluation as the district clearly had no idea how to handle the situation. Our formal request was answered with a letter of due process from the co-op. The letter of due process in essence meant that *we* were being accused of doing something out of compliance—like removing him from school (the same school that told me to take him home because they could no longer handle him!). This was all-out war. We hired an attorney and began our fight for a proper education for our son in a safe environment. After our attorney contacted the co-op, our son's aide was swiftly reassigned, without notice, and they put another in his place while waiting for our son to return to school. I had no intentions of sending Pooka back there. I couldn't even drive past the school on our way to Target without him completely losing it—and the building wasn't even visible from the road! It was a terrible feeling to see how traumatized Pooka was without knowing why. I had dreams about doing terrible things to anyone in that building who harmed my child. The school, staff, and co-op would not talk about the aide nor why he was reassigned. I felt that he might have some answer for me about what the school staff was and wasn't doing for Pooka. The only information we received was a statement that, "The problem has since been resolved." That proved guilt in my eyes as well as in our attorney's.

On the bright side, my husband was living out of state after being laid off for about six months. He was offered and took a job in Wisconsin after we realized how much better the schools were there and after we read about the state's autism waiver program. Even though we were moving out of state, our attorney wanted to pursue our case so the school would be held accountable and less likely to put another family through this. She wanted them accountable for their actions so no other kids would be harmed, be it emotionally or physically.

Our eventual move was one of the best things we ever did for Pooka. Had we known, we might have considered relocating sooner. I'll never forget the day I told Pooka that we were going to find a new house with a new school. His face lit up like I'd never seen before. He smiled and repeated, "New school." A few days later, I noticed Pooka starting to box up some of his toys. When I asked him why, he simply said, "New house."

I was scared about how things would go with the move and how Pooka would react to it all. When we finally picked the house we were going to buy, we drove three hours with Pooka and his younger brother to go see it. We really wanted the boys, especially Pooka, to see the house before we put an offer on it. We decided to walk them through three houses that day, and the one I fell in love with was the one Pooka liked the most, too.

Before we started looking at areas in and around Madison, I called each and every district I could that supposedly had a good grasp on working with kids on the spectrum. Some schools seemed confused as to why I would be calling, but quickly understood and did their best to answer my detailed questions. Some schools flat out refused to talk to us unless we could prove that we purchased a house in their district. I quickly fell in love with one district because no matter whom I spoke with, they treated me with respect, understood exactly why I was interrogating them, and *they* kept in touch with *us*! When they said they'd follow up, they meant it! We were sold and found a perfect home to go with what seemed like a great school district. Normally, I would have been skeptical, but for whatever reason, I felt peace in my heart.

The move was relatively smooth and Pooka's transition to the new home even smoother. He started summer school right away so that the staff and he could bond. He resisted in the beginning, which was really difficult for us to see. But after spending several weeks with Miss Evers, Pooka was in love with school again.

About the time when things started to go south with school back home, we opted to stop all the biomed we were doing and chose to change gears and try homeopathy. The homeopath we used did CEASE (a specific homeopathic protocol) with Pooka, and we saw some improvements with food allergies but, again, nothing significant. I kept hearing about a classical homeopath who was based in New York and took appointments over the Internet. He was highly recommended by a close autism friend of mine, and I had to get on his waiting list. In the meantime, things were going well in our new home with a new school district, and we stopped doing biomed or homeopathy with the other doctor. It was nice to not have to get Pooka to swallow a million pills or deal with some of the vials and other things the homeopath was having us do. We really started with a clean slate when we moved, and it was good.

While waiting for our appointment with the new homeopath, I was introduced to some of the other autism families he treated. There was a group of these families on Facebook who would share stories and experiences. So I joined the group to learn as much as I could and to network. Homeopathy was foreign to me. It dealt more with energy, unlike the biomedical treatments we had used in the past. The other moms helped answer my questions and gave us a renewed hope that we could reverse the damage done to our son after years of antibiotic use, vaccine damage, and food allergies. I gained sisters I never had by being a part of the group. One mom, Tex, bestowed a nickname on most of the members. After much talk about how "sweet" I was, Tex christened me with Cupcake. It all might sound silly, but I was happy for the first time in years and felt like I finally was making friends after losing so many after our son's regression. Thanks to my new sisters, I was feeling good about our future.

We really enjoyed our summer and started to relax more. Then in November 2010, we had our initial consultation with the famous "Pete the Homeopath" from New York. Boy, was that a grueling appointment. Three hours of delving deep into my soul and talking about my son. Honestly, I had no idea what I was visualizing half the time and felt almost like I was in a trance. I just kept seeing darkness and nothing else, as if I were in the deepest reaches of space where there was nothing. Just darkness. Three grueling hours later, Pete announced that our remedy was chocolate. Dear God, please tell me I didn't just waste a ton of money on some crackpot. Please!

Much to our surprise, we saw some really good results with the chocolate remedy. Pooka was as calm as he had been as a newborn. He was much more alert and seemed aware of everything around him. He even started talking better and using full sentences. One thing we didn't like was that Pooka started talking about death any time he became upset. That scared me a great deal, and we had another appointment with Pete to get to the bottom of it. After several appointments and many emails back and forth, Pete came up with another remedy that seemed to fit well. Now this, my friends, was our magic bullet!

Pooka's new remedy was hydrogen. Not only was he talking more, he was talking in complete sentences and making conversation! He would now finally ask, "Mom, what are you doing?" Be still, my heart! There was a time when Pooka didn't seem to realize that I existed. He would stare right past me. He used to throw tantrums all the time and beat me up. It devastated me year after year. I held hope that one day . . . one day . . . he would look me right in the eye and say, "I love you, Mom," and really mean it. After he switched from chocolate to hydrogen, I noticed that Pooka wanted to spend more time with me.

I was sitting on the couch, watching TV, when Pooka walked over, lifted my afghan, and snuggled in against me. I asked what he was doing, and he told me, "I'm cuddling with you." I wasn't sure how long it would last, so I didn't speak. I wanted to ask him so many questions, but I kept quiet. Pooka stayed with me for at least ten minutes. Ten minutes might not seem like much, but after waiting seven years, it felt like ten hours. Shortly after that cuddle session, I was tucking the boys in for the night and told them I loved them. Pooka looked at me with that adorable little boy smile and said, "I love you too, Mom." I gave him a firm kiss on the forehead, squeezed him tight, told him I loved him again, and scooted out the door before I lost it.

We are still so far apart, yet we're making great strides to find each other again. It's nice to swoop in for a kiss, a hug, a tickle, or just a little cuddle without Pooka recoiling and running away. It does a mama's heart good.

I still harbor a great deal of guilt. I know I did the right things at the time. I never gave up on my child, and although I pushed him, sometimes really hard, I did it with the best intentions. No one was going to tell me that my beautiful, smart boy wasn't going to grow up and amount to anything. They were dead wrong. I prayed often—to God, the gods, the universe . . . any entity that might listen and grant my wish. I still pray and feel my prayers being answered. I pray that our recovery comes sooner rather than later. I pray Pooka does well in life. I pray that he forgives me for all that I have put him through and for the times that I lost my patience with him. I pray that he will appreciate all that we've done. I'm getting my baby back, and we have some catching up to do.

MAMA BEAR'S OTHER CUBS

When I found out I was pregnant with my daughter in 1999, all was right in the world. I spent hours caressing my belly, promising her nothing but the best. I told her she could be anything she wanted to be and that I would be there to support and cheer her on every step of the way. I repeated this process when I became pregnant with my first son. I imagined how amazing it would be to watch my children grow up together and build bonds that only siblings share. When I was blessed for the third time, it was like the stars had aligned just for me. I had always dreamed of having three kids. I was one of two, and I thought having one more was absolutely ideal.

Even as a child, I recognized the special bond my brother and I shared. Even through the most vicious arguments, there was never any doubt that I had his back and he mine. I spent hours daydreaming about how each of my children's personalities would eventually mold them into the adults they would be someday. "Someday" was such a beautiful dream.

As with most families, those dreams were halted, perhaps even eternally changed, when autism came knocking on our door.

My younger son developed as a typical child. He hit all of his milestones and was the most cuddly of my three. I still feel his breath on my shoulder as he would bury his chubby cheeks into my skin and sigh. He honestly let out a sigh *every* time he rested his head on my body. It was as if he was telling me just how content he felt. He felt safe. He felt loved, and he was letting me know in his own way. But by the time he was eighteen months old, I could feel him slipping away. Eye contact became limited, he was not pointing, and his babbling and the few words he possessed came to a halt. He was sinking into his own world. As I look back on pictures, I see the emptiness in his stares and the pain in his eyes and feel the distance that was slowly pushing its way between us. He no longer felt comfortable in my arms. He would squirm and push away. He stopped sighing as he rested his head on my shoulder, and I knew at that point that our lives were about to change.

Nicholas suffered a seizure at twenty months. It was the most horrifying five minutes of my life. I found him lying by his train table. He was blue and lifeless. I handed him to my husband and ran out of the house as he began CPR on my baby. *My* baby. What happened? Why was this happening? I collapsed outside, while on the phone with 911, and all I can remember is the blood-curdling screams coming from my mouth, my soul. I began bargaining with God and asked for Him to please spare my son. I didn't know at that time whether I would ever hear him laugh, see him smile, or watch him play again. I was faced with the possibility that when I went back into my house, he would no longer be there. We joke often as parents about stressful situations taking years off our lives. This definitely did. Quite a few years were shaved off mine. When I walked back into my living room with the paramedics, Nicky was starting to come around. He was softly crying, and I could see the look of exhaustion and confusion on his beautiful little face. As the paramedics began to work on him, they realized that his eyes were pulling to the side. They then announced, "He is having a seizure." How? Why? This didn't make any sense to me. He was not convulsing; he just turned blue. The world and life I had known just moments before were now a black hole of questions and sorrow. It was swallowing me up piece by piece, moment by moment. I caught a glimpse of my daughter, Lexi, as she stood shaking and crying in the corner. I knew that she would never be the same either.

Over the next few weeks, we rushed Nick from specialist to specialist. He was scheduled for EEGs, MRIs, genetic testing, and more blood tests than I could count. In the end, all came back normal, and the doctors decided that he had a febrile seizure because the seizure was accompanied by a fever. This had to be the answer. They also stated that it was atypical in the sense that it was brought on by a sudden rise in body temperature rather than a very high fever. This did not help. I was now terrified of every cold, every sneeze, every germ that entered my home.

My daughter started kindergarten the following year, and she was thriving in every sense of the word. She was healthy and smart and had the world at her fingertips. During a class production, each child was asked to stand up in front of the room and tell the parents what they wanted to be when they grew up. I sat and watched each child make their way up to the front of the room. They were soft-spoken and shy, and some refused to speak. Most of the kids, however, announced that they wanted to be firemen, teachers, police officers, or nurses. We applauded their vision and kept snapping pictures. When it was my daughter's turn to make her way up to the front of the room, I clenched my video camera and, in true parental fashion, waited for her to say something unique and brilliant. After all, my children were special. She walked with such confidence, such poise, as she planted her little feet and smiled at me. "I am going to be a marine biologist when I grow up," she announced. Silence. Jaws were on the floor. We had never suggested anything of the sort to her. Where did she come up with this? I was in awe of her. Then it hit me. Would she ever be able to pursue such a career? Would she leave me and live far away where tropical waters surround her? Would she remain confident and follow her dreams? Or would she one day feel obligated to help her brother? What would happen to my daughter's dreams if I could no longer take care of my son? It was a bittersweet moment.

As my older son, Eric, was developing, I began to notice similar things. I wanted to offer him the world and tell him that there was nothing he couldn't do. That the world was his and I would support him in all of his ventures. Eric was different. He sensed my pain, my anxiety, and my desire to keep my kids safe and close to me. We were watching a show on TV one day, and the crew were touring mansions in various parts of the world. I looked at my son and said, "Maybe you will have a house like that one day, Eric." He smiled and replied, "No, Mommy, I am going to build a small house in our backyard and always be here for you." The tears began to roll down my face. I knew that he had been changed. Watching me over the years had stolen a part of his dreams too.

The same children who presented themselves as confident to the world were scared and worried for their little brother and parents. I remember a time when Lexi was playing innocently on the floor. Nicky had been battling a bad cold and was very tired. He stood up and stumbled a bit as I rushed to his side and began to check to see if he had a temperature. I looked in his eyes and asked if he was okay. When I realized that he was fine, I looked over my shoulder to see where the whimpering was coming from. I saw my daughter in a fetal position, rocking back and forth, covering her ears. She was sobbing. I went over to her and asked what was wrong. "Is Nicky okay, Mommy? Does he have to go to the hospital again?" I hugged her and told her that it wasn't her job to worry. She needed to leave that up to her daddy and me. I knew then that there was no way for me to protect my older kids from what was happening to their little brother . . . to me . . . to us. It was all consuming.

We all hear, at one time or another, "That's not fair," "You love him/her more," or "How come he can do that and I can't?" Sibling rivalry is an ever-present shadow that all families have dealt with over the years. It's different in our home. I hear less of it, especially when it comes to Nicky. Lexi and Eric rarely question my decisions and have accepted the fact that we are unable to do things "across the board." They are aware of their brother's limitations and do not question my love for them . . . or do they?

I was always very careful with how I divided my time. When my daughter was born, it was easy. She was to get 100 perecent of me 24/7; my only concern was her well-being and happiness. When Eric was born, I learned to split my time 50-50 for the most part. I doted on Lexi while Eric napped, and tended to his needs when she was occupied with daddy or some sort of Baby Einstein DVD. When Nicky was born, it was more of a challenge, but we always managed. I was able to care for him because Lexi and Eric would play together at that point. I would join in their fun when Nicky would nap, and they never lacked attention. We were so happy. My perfect little family was everything I had ever dreamed of and more. I had a song for each of my kids. I would sit in tears as I listened to them play and dream of the amazing people they would grow to be. I would joke about living in NJ and paying the high taxes so that they could go to amazing universities or Ivy League schools and still be close to home. Those jokes now haunt me. Will my kids stay close so that they can be here for *me*? Will they forfeit their dreams so that they can help me pick up the pieces of a life I had planned for my son? Will they feel obligated to stay in this area, even if it means altering their plans? These questions keep me awake many, many nights. I feel as if autism has robbed us all. Why, dear God, why? Why do I have to watch my children suffer? Why do I have to watch the future we once planned slip away?

Future. Such an amazing word. It is filled with hopes, dreams, goals, and the determination to get you there. When you live in a house with a child with special needs, the word *future* takes on an entirely new meaning. Most of the time, it simply means five minutes from now because you can't think beyond that. It is always about the here and now. The monotonous day by day seems to engulf your thoughts of tomorrow. You begin to say things like, "We'll see" and "I can't promise, but I'll try." You get used to seeing disappointment on their little faces because you have to cancel an outing or postpone a vacation. You are torn by the forces that pull in two very different directions. One direction is completely consumed by research and focused on finding a way to heal your sick child. The other entails striving to maintain some sort of normalcy for your neurotypical kids. I have learned to commend their efforts rather than the outcome. Although they excel as athletes as well as students, I reward their work ethics and kind hearts. While the average child is committed to impressing his or her friends, my kids have learned to be compassionate towards those who are in need. When Lexi was in second grade, her elementary school became vigilant at keeping sugar out of the classrooms. They were teaching the kids to be healthy and to be aware of the rapid rise in children with food allergies. Cupcakes to celebrate someone's birthday in the classroom became a thing of the past. My kids would occasionally come home with various toys and pencils in a goody bag. It became difficult for parents to send in food for a birthday party. When Lexi's birthday was approaching, I asked her what she wanted to do. Without any hesitation she said, "I want to donate the money you would spend on cupcakes or goody bags to kids with autism." I couldn't believe it. My baby girl, at the tender age of seven, was completely selfless. She printed up an article on autism and read it to her class. She then gave them each a thank-you card that stated that a donation had been made in their class's name. I still tear up thinking about it. The organization to which they donated sent them a certificate that their teacher proudly displayed on a classroom wall. A few days after the "party," I got a phone call from a parent, whose son was in Lexi's class. She proceeded to tell me that her son came home excited and told her all about what he had learned in school that day. He told her that he knew what autism was and that his class was helping kids who suffer from the disorder. She was so thrilled and said that there had never been mention, in past years, of how delicious a cupcake was or how much he liked a pencil or eraser he had received. Lexi had managed to touch a child. She had educated a group of children that will one day be our future. Maybe that is what we need to focus on when we say *future*.

Recently, I overheard Lexi talking to her friends about her little brothers. She stated that although Eric drives her crazy, he will always be her little buddy. She then went on to say that Nicky had Asperger's but was the smartest little boy she knew. She bragged about his ability to memorize things like no one else can and how he navigates the Internet with ease. She joked about how all her friends adore him and have adopted him as their little brother as well. She has grown into the spectacular young lady I always knew she would be.

Eric has matured as well. He often refers to Nicky as his "best friend" and talks about how strong and amazing his little brother is. He notices and points out gains and will always congratulate each of Nicky's accomplishments. He takes his little brother on the trampoline and allows him to dictate the games they will play. He puts his own needs aside and never questions why Nicky may have taken the last ice-cream sandwich. Eric is an old soul with the heart of a lion tucked neatly inside the body of a nine-year-old boy.

While most parents discuss light-hearted, grandiose plans with their children, we talk about deeper things. We talk about what would happen if my husband and I were not around. We talk about how to treat the people around us. We talk about the importance of family and all that it stands for. They tell me that they will always look out for their little brother and make sure that he is taken care of. It's not what I want to talk about, but I have to say that I am extremely proud of them. They have become exactly what I had hoped for and more. I am confident now that they will be successful. The terrible, tragic, scary, and painful things that autism brought to us have also helped us to become better people. We fight for the rights of those who need our help. We cry for those whose lives are tormented by this pain. We have learned to be compassionate. We have learned to be a little more human. All the things that autism stole from us have been replaced with new dreams, new hopes, and knowledge. Maybe my daughter will not become a marine biologist, but she may become a social worker, or an attorney who takes on malpractice suits. Or maybe, just maybe, she'll be an amazing stay-at-home mom who is a little more patient and a little more attentive to her children's needs. Maybe my son will stay close to home and remain loyal to his roots. Maybe he will become a pediatrician, maybe a blue-collar worker, maybe a judge. Whatever they choose to be *when they grow up*, I know that they will be amazing people.

The word *future* is an ever-changing term here. Some days, it seems like it's a million miles away. Other days, it seems as if it presents itself to us in clear fashion. We treat it as the most delicate of words, and we cherish its meaning. The future means healing my son and watching him become the man he was intended to be. The future means leaving no stone unturned and remaining hopeful for each of my children. The future has allowed us to learn from our past, embrace the present, and put our faith in a better tomorrow . . . even if it is just one day at a time.

TEX: AN EXCAVATION OF SPIRITUAL AUTISM IN ONE ACT

Lights go down on an empty stage. Suddenly and without warning, a single spotlight shines abruptly on a slender, tallish, ethnically ambiguous female standing center stage. She seemingly appeared out of nowhere. Shielding her eyes as she glances toward the spotlight above, she blinks, trying to get her bearings. Her unruly curly hair is held out of her face by a printed scarf folded into a headband. Untamed hair. Unkempt clothes. And an almost failed attempt at "hip" that strangely seems to work for her. She wears her heart on her sleeve. She's a fighter. Today, her uncertainties are reflected in her softness. There's casualness about her visage and a panic in her nature.

TEX: Hello? <no answer> Hello??? Uhmmm . . . Hi??? <silence>
    It's me—Tex? I think you were expecting me? <more silence>
    I had an appointment, right? Hello??
<a look of confusion comes over her face; she's slightly shaken and uncomfortable>

TEX: Sorry. Do you mind if we talk out loud? I find the whole "in your head" thing . . . it's weird. Know what I mean? I'm a little freaked out. I mean—it's totally your call, but I'm trippin'. Just a little.

VOICE: <*sounding strangely like James Earl Jones*> Better?

TEX: Better. And thanks for choosing a nice big booming God voice. It really helps. I just don't need any more paradigm shifts right now. <*she laughs nervously*> Okay—well—thanks for agreeing to see me. Or hear me or whatever cuz I can't see you and I can only hear you, but you can probably see and hear me and feel me and everything so it's hard to know . . . okay . . . well . . . okay I just want you to know I appreciate your time.

VOICE: I know.

TEX: Well alrighty then. So—I'll just cut right to the chase . . . I'm here cuz . . . well you know why I'm here, don't you? You know everything, right? You knew I was coming, and you know about my life and how bad things suck sometimes and how I wish I could go back and change things and well . . . about my son's autism. <*silence*> Cuz that's why I'm here. You know I'm here because of him, right? I mean—I'm super cool with the big questions in life—I don't need to fully understand you or why you've designed things the way you have or why bad things happen to good people and stuff like that—I mean, my faith is enough for most things. It really is. I don't have a ton of questions. You know that. You know I've never asked, and I've been super accepting and stoked to be able to love you and hang out with you. Heck—I call you J-dad. In so many ways . . . you're my daddy. I'm totally into you. But you know why I'm here. Right? You know. You know that on this one subject I struggle. I need to reconcile being totally into you and understanding . . . You know . . . understanding . . .

<*long pause*>

TEX: <*she chokes on the next word*> Why.

<*silence*>

TEX: <*she's steeled herself*> So why?

<*silence*>

VOICE: Why.

TEX: *Oh. Em. Gee.* By "gee" I mean gosh. Not . . . okay, whatever. <*hurt more than angry*> Seriously, Pops? Did you just ask
me why why??? Really? Okay, so you didn't really ask—you
just repeated the word, but it kind of puts the ball back in
my court right?

    I did everything right. You know that. I breastfed, I did
organic baby food, I delayed the vaccines for goodness sake.
But you knew—he had that hypospadias, and you knew we
would correct it and he would have surgery at twelve months
old and he would never be the same after that, and you knew
and you knew and *you knew.* And why? *Why? Why* did he
have to be the one? Why not me? Why not keep me from
making kids at all? Cuz this sucks monkey turds. It really does,
Dad. Why would you put me through this, why? <*she struggles
to regain her composure*>

<*pause*>

TEX: Okay—I get it. It's not the end of the world. And there are
people in much worse situations. I get it. I just . . . Would
you say something, please?

<*pause*>

VOICE: <*the voice now sounds more like a loving dad and less like James
Earl Jones*> You know I love you?

TEX: Yes. I know you do. I really know it.

VOICE: How do you know?

TEX: *Ha!* I ask my kids the same question all the time. Well . . .
Trinity anyway. Okay. I'll play. I know because you don't
leave me. No matter what I do. No matter how awful I am or
how much I screw things up—you're always there. You show
up in the most amazing ways. You never give up on me. It's
like with the twins—no matter what they do, no matter how
angry they may make me—I love them. I always love them,
and that love doesn't change. You love me like that. I guess

that's what's so confusing—you love me so much, and you
did this to my son.

VOICE: It's not of my making.

TEX: No. I suppose it isn't. <*clearly saddened*> We're in an imperfect world run by imperfect men doing imperfect things.
And so . . . is it random? Did you choose him or me randomly? Was this just bad luck? You could prevent things,
you know.

VOICE: I could.

TEX: But then you'd be negating the whole free will thing and
natural consequences blah blah blah . . . I get it. The human
race has done this. It's a toxic world with toxic people, and
there are bound to be consequences. Is there a point? Was
I chosen or something? Is there a reason?

VOICE: Do you trust me?

TEX: <*thinks*> Yes. Yes. Actually I do. And I see how you've
allowed this to shape me. I see how much more aware and
mature I've become. I also see how much closer we are.
I need you more. We're better friends. You're not so . . .
distant anymore. I see the good that comes of struggle. I do.
I trust you. It's just that . . . I miss his eyes. You know?
You remember? Remember that day he was like what, three
months old?

VOICE: Four.

TEX: Four months old—and he looked up at me from the crib.
<*her voice goes into almost a monotone*> That blue Winnie the
Pooh sheet was on the mattress. The one I bought from
Target. Trinity had a matching beige one over on her crib,
and Lance had the blue one. And he looked up at me and
laughed and smiled and held my eyes for the longest . . . <*her
voice trails*> and I thought to myself, *He has the best sense of
humor. Why doesn't Trinity smile and laugh as much as he does?*
<*she tries in vain to shake it off*> So yes. I trust you. But I miss
him. I miss that feeling . . . like we were connected . . . I miss
the magic you gave us in that moment. <*she pleads in a raspy
deep voice that reflects the depths of her passion; all pretense is*

gone> Please . . . Please . . . Please . . . *Please,* can I just have
that again? Please? Just once . . . *<she is almost panting>* I'll
do anything. Anything. Just once more. Like that. Like that
day. Please.

<silence>

TEX: *<she loses it>* You know what? *Fuck you. Fuck you!!!!* You
could do it. You could take it away. *You could fucking do
it!!!!!! What the fuckity fuck fuck fuck are you waiting for!?!?!?!?!?
Fuck you fuck you fuck you fuck fuck fuck fuck fuck!!!!!!!!!! <she
sinks to the ground sobbing>*

*<a good long cry and a heart-wrenching moan from the depths of another
dimension play out until finally she is done; the tears are gone, and she
is spent; there is nothing; she stares into space with an almost childlike
innocence>*

TEX: I did this. I did. I brought this on him. That night in the restaurant in Ashland, Oregon. We were at dinner with Mike's
parents. I was what? Seven months pregnant?

VOICE: Eight.

TEX: *<chuckles>* Eight. And my sweet, precious, perfect mother-
in-law told me the most important thing was that the twins
be healthy. She told me to pray for their health. And I had
the audacity to argue with her. You remember? I said, "Is it?
Is that really the most important thing? Because there are
lots of healthy people who are unhappy. I mean, if one of
the kids were born with a heart defect or autism . . ." *Ha!!!!*
I used the word autism. I did. I told her that I would be able
to handle it as long as they were happy and loved Jesus. *<her
voice cracks>* I said that. I did. You heard me. You heard me,
and you let it happen like I had wished it on him. I was so
self-righteous and proud of myself for my amazing spiritual
insight. Oh. Em. Gee. And this time . . . I mean, oh my God.
My sweet precious Lord. Tell me I didn't do this. Please. Tell
me I'm wrong.

<a small pause>

VOICE: *<with the utmost tenderness>* You're wrong.

<she smiles as tears roll down her face; a huge burden has been lifted>

TEX: <*she prays out loud as she kneels*> Oh, sweet Jesus. Thank you. Thank you for that. Thank you. And thank you—thank you for that moment. Thank you for the blue Winnie the Pooh sheet. Thank you. Thank you for giving me that. So precious. So precious. Thank you. Thank you for letting him talk and walk and do the things his sister did right alongside her. Thank you. Thank you, thank you, thank you, thank you for that first year. Oh, God, thank you. <*she is overwhelmed with gratitude and joy—the tears continue to roll*> And thank you for giving me twins. Oh, thank you. Thank you for giving them to each other and to me, and thank you. And how do I thank you? How do I thank you for my precious, precious babies? Sweet Jesus, thank you.

<*silence as she finishes her quiet cry and comes to peace*>

TEX: Sorry I said the *F* word.

VOICE: <*now sounds like a matronly woman*> It's not the first time I've heard it.

<*she laughs*>

TEX: No. I suppose it isn't. Still. You're God and all. I should have more respect. The word is offensive.

VOICE: The word doesn't offend me. People's hearts offend me.

<*silence*>

TEX: My anger didn't offend you?

VOICE: Your *pain* didn't offend me.

TEX: Oh, God, I love you.

VOICE: And I love you.

TEX: I know. I'm so glad. I really am. So glad and grateful. So glad you're my J-dad. <*pause*>

You remember it, right? World Autism Day. April 2, 2008. The day I became <*she signals quotes signs in the air*> aware. I'll never forget that day, you know. CNN was running a million stories about autism and the vaccine controversy. Back then, it was a controversy. Now they say it's a myth. They play God, you know. They try to improve on the immune system, the food, the environment . . . they make it all toxic. Chemicals. And then they wonder why the kids are full of allergies and have asthma. Obesity, diabetes, . . . autism. But it's a myth? No. It's no myth. Lance came out of that surgery room a completely different child.

He was so angry. The screaming and crying. The way he'd tense his whole body like a board. And you were there, right? You were there when I took the baby spoon from the drawer. It had that blue coating on the spoon head, and I took it and dug rock-hard poop from his butt. He was screaming and crying, and I was crying, and Mike stood over us horrified. But what could I do? The baby was in so much pain and so blocked up, and so I dug. I dug shit out of his ass. Rock-hard, horrible shit pellets from hell. I dug and dug and dug until diarrhea shot out behind the rocks of crap. And I was covered in it. We were all covered in it. We still are. We're still trying to dig the crap out and find my son again. It's what we have to do. Dig. <*she stops and thinks*>

<*she's numb, and her voice reflects it*> If anesthesia can trigger autism—and it did—vaccines can, too. I'm right, aren't I? All these chronic diseases and illnesses—heart disease, cancer, Alzheimer's, all the autoimmune disorders—all these things are on the rise because we're trying to play God. We've taken you out of our lives and our hearts and our food and our world. We can't even see you anymore for the skyscrapers and smog. And this is the price. This is the price for turning away.

VOICE: <*James Earl Jones is back*> Yes.

TEX: When he was fourteen months . . .

VOICE: <*interrupts*> Sixteen.

TEX: Sixteen.

When he was sixteen months, he was hitting those children at that women's bible study I used to host. Remember? I don't know why I keep asking you if you remember. I know you remember. <*sighs*> Anyway . . . I remember telling Mike that night I thought Lance was a sociopath. Mike thought I was crazy. But I did. I thought we had some kind of psychotic sociopath on our hands. He was just so disconnected. He didn't care about anyone. He just walked around hitting kids for no reason. He wasn't even mad. He was just . . . mean. Mean and uncaring. But not with a mean purpose. With a nothing purpose. He was scary. I was scared. I was scared of my sixteen-month-old baby. I was scared of him because the baby he had been was gone and this . . . this . . . automaton was left here instead. And then . . . after that . . . I couldn't understand you and me anymore. I was doing things the way I thought you wanted me to. I was going to church and praying and looking for you and talking with you. But maybe . . . maybe that was a good thing that I lost my way? Because back then you seemed so far away and unreal. You were so . . . God-like. And now . . . now that I'm unclear and unsure and so lost—now . . . now you're . . . accessible? Approachable? Your voice even changes to suit what I need. Holy *cow*— I can even walk up to you like this. Just like this. I can do this. I can do what I'm doing. I can say the *F* word at you and scream at you and be with you, and you're real. You're really, really real. Were you really, really real before? Really?

<*realizations continue to ensue*> I get it. I do. I am so sorry. Oh, dear God. Please forgive me. I am so, so, so sorry. I know you've been reaching out. I feel you. I feel you trying to put your arms around me. I feel you trying so hard to communicate. I don't know why I turn away. I don't know why I give you the spiritual bird. You ask me to talk to you, and I don't. I don't pray. I don't chat. I thought I was doing all those things when you were some kind of distant unattainable burning bush in the sky. But I wasn't. Not really. Our relationship wasn't a relationship at all. How friggin' ironic is that? Oh . . . but the irony just continues to grow. Because now . . . now that I can actually *feel* you carrying me and holding my hand and reaching out . . . Now I turn my back. Now I try to do everything my way.

I ask for things, and you tell me to wait or you don't give me an answer, and I throw a fit. It's like with my kids—I tell them to eat their peas first because I have ice cream waiting for them, but all they can see is the piece of gum they want right now. <*slow realization*> I have spiritual autism, don't I? You call my name, and I don't respond. I can't listen or focus. I'm too distracted by my own agenda to listen or hear you. I live in my own little bubble. I tune you out. I do my own thing. I hurt people. I hurt myself. I'm disobedient and willful and defiant. I perseverate on Facebook and my text messages. I have spiritual autism. <*she tries to control a sob*> I have spiritual autism.

VOICE: <*loving dad is back*> Most people do.

TEX: What's the therapy?

VOICE: Me. More me.

TEX: I'm recoverable?

VOICE: <*matron mama*> Managed recovery.

TEX: Okay. Managed recovery. You're the manager? Okay. I like that. I can do that. It takes the pressure off. And Lance . . . I almost asked "what about Lance" . . .

    I came here to ask "Why," but I should be asking "How?" It's about focusing on *how* to give him more of you as well, isn't it? Recovery. How. Those are my two words. You've given me so many things to help him. I know it's the toxicity. He's full of metals and nasties, and it's causing yeast, and bacteria are attacking his little brain, and there are probably viruses. His gut can't handle the man-made, processed junk most people are eating these days. <*she's discovering her answers*> We need to get back to *you*. You've provided the food he needs, the medicine. Organic food. Frequent low-dose chelation. Supplements to support his deficiencies. Herbs. Therapies. Human connection. You've given us what we need to help him. You have.

    Okay, okay, okay. I can do this. I'm a bit blown away right now. I mean, it's one thing to know this stuff, but it's another thing to really *know* it. <*she pauses and reflects*> You really are everything. Creator. Healer. Author. Redeemer. Father. Friend . . . J-dad. I didn't need to come here to figure this out, did I? You've been trying to tell me all of this all along. You know . . . this pretty much sucks. It does. I don't like all this work, and I don't like seeing my son in pain. I hate what this does to his sister and my marriage. I hate it. But you hate it too. You do. You're in more pain than I am because you feel our pain and everyone else's too. This isn't what you wanted or what you planned. And some day, things will be different. You'll fix it. You'll fix it all. This whole stupid world, it'll be gone, and you'll make everything all better. You will.

VOICE: <*James Earl*> It won't be long.

TEX: *Ha!!!* Relative to what? Not long for you seems to be a gazillion lifetimes to the rest of us. But what about Lance? How long will it take for him? You know . . . to get better?

VOICE: <*matron mama*> That depends. He is loved. He loves. He is taught. He teaches. He is challenged. He challenges. He touches your heart, and you touch his. But it isn't only you he touches. He touches the world around him. He ministers. He does my work. He is my hands and feet. He is my heart. He has work to do, and so do you. I always provide blessings in the challenges. The question is . . . can you find those blessings? Can you live in them? Can you be strong in them and allow them to help you get through the struggles? Can you use the blessings to help you dig?

   I promise to provide all he needs to continue to progress. It's up to you to find and utilize that provision. Take care of him and his darling sister. I've entrusted them to you, and your job is to care for them and lead them back to me. Teach them that their bodies are temples, and help them open their hearts so I can take up residence there. That is your purpose.

VOICES: <*all three voices at the same time*> Love them and teach them to love. It's what I am after all. Faith, hope, and love, but the greatest of these is love. Love. Your faith and hope are worthless without it.

<*long pause*>

TEX: Love. So simple. So simple. So complicated. So "you." Okay. I can do that. And I can trust. I can just trust. At least, I can right now, in this moment. But that doesn't mean I'm not gonna freak out again from time to time.

<*pause*>

TEX: Thank you. Thank you for doing this with me. Thank you for putting up with my autism. I used to think it would be such a special thing to be able to come to you like this. I was so stupid. I didn't realize—I've always been able to come to you like this. And I can. Any day. Any time. You're there. You're really there.

<*something catches her eye; she looks down at the ground and picks something up in front of her feet; she holds up a little baby spoon with blue coating*>

<*a single sob escapes her, but she quickly steels herself; she wipes her eyes with the back of her hand and stares straight forward with purpose; a slow smile emerges as her face fortifies into pure confidence; she appears to grow two inches taller; she is suddenly sexy and wild and bright; she appears to glow; it becomes almost blinding to look at her; she is intimidating and confident as she speaks with a slow quiet authority . . .* >

TEX: Okay. Time to dig.

<*spotlight goes out abruptly*>

Bytes from the Count

I'm jittery, I'm nervous. I look at the calendar, flip through the months. Panic sets in. Time is going by, and I need progress. Every birthday that goes by, I die a little more inside.

DRAGON SLAYER BEYOND BORDERS: A TALE OF TWO RECOVERIES

Mummy, are you going to America to visit Justin Bieber?

I was packing for a week-long trip to Chicago to attend the Autism-One/Generation Rescue Conference, not looking forward to the twenty-seven-hour flight from Kuala Lumpur, the multiple layovers, and jetlag. My daughters, Mei and Min Min, were playing dress up, trying on my clothes and shoes. I stopped, smiling at Mei's question, and replied, "No, I'm going there to learn and study hard." She was silent for a while, her face serious. I jokingly asked if she wanted to marry Justin Bieber, because last week she told me she wanted to marry Aladdin. The month before, she wanted to marry Prince Charming. Mei immediately replied, "No, I want to show Justin Bieber my pet goldfish!" Min Min then started singing "Baby, baby, baby, oooohh!" at the top of her lungs, and off the two girls went, singing and dancing away. A couple of years ago, I couldn't have imagined such a typical scene.

In 2008, Mei was diagnosed with moderate autism. One year later, my younger daughter, Min Min, too, started regressing. She was two years old and rapidly spiraling down the path into autism. Since then, in an effort to heal my daughters, I have attended autism biomedical conferences in Singapore, Bangkok, Hong Kong, and several major cities in the United States. I have consulted with doctors in Singapore, Indonesia, Australia, United Kingdom, and America. I would travel to the ends of the earth if I had to. Nothing would stop me from recovering my girls from autism . . . After all, what's an ocean between me and recovery, right?

This is an autism recovery story that crosses borders, spanning countries, ethnicities, and cultures. This is my Malaysian tale.

Cast of characters:

Mei: Loves fairies, unicorns, rainbows, and pink. Her greatest wish is to go to Disneyland. Wants to grow up to be a mermaid and marry Prince Charming.

Min Min: Loves sparkly shoes, purple, dressing up in mummy's clothes, and bossing her big sister around. My glitter punk princess. Her ambition is to be a pirate princess.

Hubby (aka Poop Smuggler): Patient husband, father of two, and frequent-flyer businessman. Sydneysider who cracks Australian jokes. The sole voice of reason.

Me (aka Dragon Slayer): Autism advocate. Adores shoes, handbags, and sci-fi/fantasy. Runs on coffee, hot bird's-eye chili, and spicy curries. Earth mother goddess wannabe.

Hubby is a blue-eyed Australian who grew up in the surfs of Bondi Beach. When we met, he had just been transferred to Kuala Lumpur, the capital of Malaysia—a modern city with a laid-back vibe. I had grown up in a small Malaysian village and gone to work in the big city. We had a "big fat Malaysian wedding" in Kuala Lumpur, attended by his family from Australia, friends from all over the world, and my Malaysian family and friends. We were in love, we were happy, and we wanted children—preferably girls to dress up in pink and frilly clothes and go shoe shopping with.

My first pregnancy was easy, not even a day of morning sickness. Because the baby was breech, I had a cesarean birth—a pain- and stress-free experience. Mei was born on a gorgeous spring morning in Sydney, Australia. With such a breezy pregnancy and an equally serene birth, we were gobsmacked when the reality of raising Mei was not the laid-back experience we had envisioned it would be.

From the day she was born, Mei hardly ever slept and had difficulty latching on to breastfeed. She had terrible colic and reflux and screamed nonstop for four to six hours every night. She slept one to two hours at a stretch, and her face was covered with red, scaly rashes. At three weeks, Mei was diagnosed with bilateral hip dysplasia. She was placed in a Pavlick harness, to be worn for twenty-four hours a day for at least three months. We moved back to Kuala Lumpur soon after. The confines of the restrictive harness, combined with the tropical heat in Malaysia, made her a very unhappy baby. Those few months went by in a haze of screaming and crying.

She had twelve bowel movements a day, the poop shooting out of her little bum so hard it squirted out of her nappy. Often she would be covered from neck to toe in her own poop. Hubby turned out to be an incredible hands-on father, patiently cleaning her up for the umpteenth time. This went on for months. We went to the doctor often, returning with prescriptions for colic medication, steroid creams, and yet more antibiotics for her constant colds and flu.

I loved my beautiful, exotic daughter deeply, but I never imagined raising a baby would be this difficult; after all, none of my family or friends ever had such a fussy baby. All the other babies I knew were contented little angels, not like this red-faced, screaming, projectile-vomiting, miserable little girl with rocket-trajectory poops.

Nonetheless, both our Malaysian and Australian pediatricians declared her to be "normal." Mei hit all her developmental milestones on time. I treasure the photographs and videos of her when she was younger, brimming with life and enthusiasm. Before the shining light and the depth of her soul in her eyes dimmed, before she turned into a shadow of her true self. Before autism took away so much of her joy and happiness.

Apart from her constant whining, fussiness, and tantrums, I thought everything was fine. It never occurred to me that she never called me Mummy. Nor did she ever request anything. If she wanted something, she would scream in a tantrum until I figured out what she wanted. Or she would take my hand and point it to the item she wanted. Deep inside, I felt that I was a failure as a mother.

Like every good parent, I took my daughter for her vaccinations. Since Mei is Australian and we would be living in Malaysia, we thought it would be a good idea to follow the vaccination schedule of both countries for double protection. More is surely better than less, right? She got her hep B, DTP, MMR, and other shots, including the BCG for tuberculosis, as per the Malaysian vaccine schedule.

Though Mei was a difficult and fussy child, we loved her so much that we wanted another baby just like her. So we decided to have a second child as soon as possible, and we were pleased when I got pregnant when Mei was seven months old. We moved back to Sydney a few months before my due date. Min Min was born when Mei was one and a half. At that time, Mei was a bright, happy little girl. She was sociable, engaging, and intelligent. Though she had not progressed to making proper conversation, she still labeled a lot and had some nonverbal communication skills. Probably due to the haze of my pregnancy, and later the adrenaline high from Min Min's birth, I only saw the glowing, happy big sister Mei was.

In Sydney, Mei got the meningococcal C vaccine as required under the Australian vaccination schedule. I was still recovering from Min Min's birth and was at home nursing her when my husband took Mei to the health center in North Sydney. He came home with Mei still sobbing in his arms. He said she'd screamed the place down when the nurse administered the shot. That turned out to be her last vaccine.

We moved back to Kuala Lumpur with two beautiful little girls. We seemed like the perfect family, but in reality, life was anything but perfect. Raising Mei was extremely challenging. In contrast, Min Min was a happy, contented, and easygoing baby from the day she was born. She slept most of the time and was a joy to be with. It only then occurred to me that *this* was what a normal baby is like. It was my first inkling that our troubles with Mei were abnormal, that perhaps I was not such a terrible mother after all, that perhaps something else made raising Mei such an ordeal.

Despite having a full-time nanny, a maid, and my parents around to help, we were struggling mightily with Mei. She was uncontrollable, her rages and tantrums legendary. Five adults could not control her. Whenever she cried, which was often, it sounded as if she were being tortured. We hardly went out, because Mei would scream if she were in a strange place. She would have an epic meltdown if we went to a noisy restaurant. Mei would wrench herself free from my grasp and run into the street into oncoming traffic. She was scared of men, especially tall or dark-skinned men, something pretty hard to avoid living in multicultural Malaysia. We ceased to socialize. We were living in a cocoon in which we tried to keep Mei wrapped up in a cotton-wool world: a world with no crowds, loud noises, or bright lights.

Mei started to regress. She spoke less and less and became echolalic, repeating meaningless phrases again and again. She would often laugh out loud at inappropriate times. She no longer responded when we called her. We used to worry that Mei would get envious of her new baby sister. Instead, Mei hardly ever noticed the baby. She walked on tiptoe—spinning, running around in circles, and looking out of the corner of her eyes. She had auditory and visual processing disorders, causing her to cry out in agony over certain noises and lights. She slept badly. She was hyperactive and frequently mouthed and licked things. She would scratch until her skin bled, pull out clumps of her hair, or lie down and bang her head repeatedly on the hard floor. She would hit her head so hard, I was scared her skull would break.

We noticed Mei's behavior was worse on days she was constipated, which was often. When we mentioned our concerns to our pediatrician, all we got were more prescriptions for laxatives with no long-term solution offered. The stress, frustration, and exhaustion were taking a huge toll on us. We had a lot of unanswered questions. Doctor after doctor told us that Mei was fine, that I was an overanxious mother, and that I surfed the Internet too much. Our pediatrician said, "She will grow out of it."

Unsatisfied, I kept reading and researching. I found nothing that gave me a clue to why Mei behaved this way until Jenny McCarthy's *Louder Than Words* initially arrived in Malaysia. I had been a fan of Jenny's books ever since her first book, *Belly Laughs*. I expected an entertaining diversion, a little bit of humor to inject into my gray, turbulent life. Instead, the book changed our lives. In order to snatch a few minutes to read, I would hide in the bathroom between breastfeeding Min Min and dealing with Mei's latest meltdown. With every chapter I read, a growing sense of dread built up in me. I felt my heart crumple with every symptom of her son, Evan, that Jenny wrote about. By the end of the book, I knew in the deepest recesses of my tired old soul that Mei had autism, too.

Mei was finally diagnosed with moderate autism—after being assessed by a developmental pediatrician, a clinical psychologist, and a child psychiatrist in Kuala Lumpur—at two years eight months.

At first, the diagnosis brought relief; we finally knew what was wrong. We could start finding appropriate therapies and treatments. But soon, panic rose as the enormity of the situation sank in. We were advised to put Mei on a lifetime of psychotropic medications and prepare to institutionalize her when she was older. When asked about dietary intervention or nutritional supplements, the doctor told us to feed her more *ikan bilis*, a type of small dried anchovies. Seriously? Needless to say, Hubby and I refused to accept that this would be Mei's fate.

I was inspired by Jenny McCarthy and her son Evan's journey to recovery. As a way to motivate myself, I would say, "If Jenny can do it, so can I." Jenny had great improvement with a GFCF (gluten-free, casein-free) diet. The more I read about it, the more I knew it would be beneficial for Mei. Always a picky eater, Mei would happily eat bread and cookies all day if we let her. And she was absolutely addicted to milk. Hubby and I used to joke about how woozy Mei would get after drinking a full bottle of milk, as if she were drunk or high on drugs. We put her on the diet the day she was diagnosed. Fortunately, going GFCF in Malaysia was relatively easy, as most of Malaysian cuisine does not contain wheat and dairy. Within the first week, Mei uttered her first request; she looked me in the eye and said, "Milk." This skill would come and go but was encouraging, nonetheless. In the meantime, I put together a team of therapists for applied behavior analysis (ABA), one of the few behavioral therapies available in Malaysia at that time. We were overjoyed to see her respond well, making slow but steady progress. There were no biomedical doctors in Malaysia at the time, and I didn't feel I could justify the extra expense of traveling to another country. So, I decided to pursue biomedical treatments for Mei on my own. Unfortunately, my methods were haphazard, and Mei did not show the improvements I had hoped.

In the midst of all this, Min Min grew into a healthy, happy toddler with the sweetest disposition. She showered me with kisses and hugs, and in turn, I lavished her with all the pent-up love and affection that I was unable to lavish on Mei. Though I knew it was because of autism, I still felt crushed every time Mei rejected my overtures of love. Min Min soothed my broken heart in more ways than I could imagine.

I nearly burst into tears when Min Min called me Mummy for the first time. I had waited three years for Mei to call me Mummy. Even then, it was another year before she did it spontaneously. I lapped up every word Min Min said. Eventually, she went on to acquire more expressive language; she was advanced for her age.

A few months after Mei's diagnosis, we took a much-needed holiday and spent a few days at a lovely resort in Phuket, Thailand. One day, Hubby took the girls to play under the lawn sprinklers. A couple of the gardeners yelled at them in Thai, then another member of the staff ran up to us and kindly translated. It turns out the sewage system had just broken down, and sewage had seeped into the sprinkler system. We quickly bathed the children and didn't give it another thought till we got home and both girls got severely ill with rotavirus. They were hospitalized for three days each, one after the other. I slept on the floor every single night, unwilling to leave them. I spent the time reading more about biomedical treatments and came to the conclusion that I needed the help of an experienced biomedical doctor to guide us on this long journey.

The girls recovered fairly quickly. Soon after they were discharged, I flew to Singapore with Hubby and Mei to consult with what turned out to be the first of many helpful biomedical practitioners. Mei showed slow but steady progress under the guidance of our first doctor. But, after a few months, I decided to consult another biomedical doctor, again based in Singapore. The second doctor, Dr. E, helped a great deal and is our primary doctor to this day. Mei responded very well to nutritional supplements, probiotics, antifungals, and antivirals. Methyl donors were excellent for her; we saw huge improvements on MB12 and TMG. The supplements are too many to list here, but suffice it to say, the progress we saw made all the effort to purchase the supplements worthwhile.

We had to send urine and stool samples to the doctor in Singapore. After finally obtaining clean samples, I stored the specimens carefully in the containers provided. I packed them with ice packs and packaged them up properly. For three days, I walked around with the parcel in my favorite designer handbag. I went to several courier companies, pleading with them to send it to Singapore. I even obtained a special shipment declaration and a letter from our doctor, but I kept getting rejected. No one wanted to deliver pee and poop. The samples have a time limit on viability, and time was running out. Hubby jumped to the rescue and volunteered to deliver them himself. He got on the next flight to Singapore, carrying a small bag loaded with urine and stool. Cool as a cucumber, he strolled past security checkpoints in the Malaysia and Singapore airports. A risky solution, but the stakes were high. He would do anything for his little girl, even smuggle pee and poop. Since then, I've looked at him with awe—my heroic Poop Smuggler! (To this day, I swear that handbag still stinks after the humiliation it was subjected to. Note to self: Treat couture with respect.)

Mei was thriving and progressing due to a combination of ABA therapy and intensive biomedical intervention, but Min Min took longer to recover from the rotavirus. She alternated between constipation and diarrhea, her stomach frequently bloated, and she lost her appetite. Though she retained most of her language skills, we noticed her development had plateaued. Most glaringly, our previously sweet and gentle Min Min was constantly throwing tantrums. Every little thing would set her off. Every week, her behavior deteriorated, and her tantrums and meltdowns were grim and frightening. It all seemed so horribly familiar.

It got to the point where Mei, our "officially diagnosed" daughter was slightly easier to manage than Min Min, our "neurotypical" daughter. Whatever language skills Min Min still had left were overshadowed by her increasingly difficult behavior. She started walking on tiptoe and became fixated on spinning objects. Min Min was hyperactive, noncompliant, and out of control. She, too, started having difficulty sleeping. She bit everyone in sight, especially her big sister, Mei, who was still too lost in her own world to notice when she was injured. Mei didn't know how to retaliate or even defend herself. Oh, how Min Min tormented her big sister! We tried our best to protect both girls, but frequently I felt that it was more than I could handle. The rotavirus had caused even more damage than we initially thought. With sinking hearts, my husband and I agreed that Min Min was also spiraling down into autism.

We chose not to seek a formal diagnosis for Min Min, mainly because it was expensive. We decided we would rather use the money to treat her than get a label du jour. Furthermore, we didn't need a piece of paper to tell us what we already knew in our hearts: Min Min was on the autism spectrum. We now had two children on the spectrum. How did life turn out like this? Needless to say, my husband and I were devastated. Raising two daughters on the autism spectrum was taking a severe toll on us, both physically and mentally. I have incredible respect for Kim Stagliano, legendary managing editor of the *Age of Autism*, who is raising three daughters on the spectrum and blazing a trail in the autism community.

We started Min Min on biomedical treatments. By that time, we could not afford behavioral therapy for Min Min. Unlike her older sister who seemed to progress in leaps and bounds, Min Min's recovery was slower. There were many stops and starts, many unsuccessful treatments, and too little progress to show for the amount of money and effort we put in. Min Min alternated between constipation and diarrhea. Eventually, she had chronic diarrhea, which lasted nine months. An x-ray revealed a serious fecal impaction. After persistent gut pain, mucousy diarrhea, and a particularly nasty rash, Min Min had an endoscopy and colonoscopy in Kuala Lumpur. The scope revealed nothing. I wondered whether we would have found signs of inflammation and lesions if we had done the procedure in another country. The doctor ruled out colitis and instead diagnosed Min Min with irritable bowel syndrome.

Though initially disheartened because the scope did not shed new light on Min Min's condition, we continued with biomedical treatments. With strict dietary restrictions and intensive biomedical treatment, Min Min's behavior slowly improved. Treatments for clostridia overgrowth, gut dysbiosis, digestive disorders, and immune modulators made a huge difference in her. She became calmer, and her violent mood swings receded. We could finally see some progress in her development. She was finally ready for school, and I enrolled her in kindergarten. Initially, she screamed and cried when we brought her there, but eventually she grew comfortable with her new teachers. In school, she finally learned to socialize and improve her communication skills.

We were seeing glimpses of recovery, and each day brought more healing. The girls were both progressing. I no longer feared that they would regress back into the depths of autism. I could feel us slowly but surely moving away from the gravitational pull of autism and all its horrors.

Eventually, we transitioned Mei into a mainstream kindergarten with the help of a shadow aide. By mid 2010, Mei no longer required specialized one-on-one ABA therapy. She then went on to two other kindergartens. Finally, in the third and last kindergarten, Mei found her groove. She no longer required an aide, and

I chose not to inform the school of Mei's diagnosis. Mei did really well there. She honed her social skills and made friends. She learned to read, write, and do math. A couple of years earlier, she could barely speak English; now Mei is learning to speak Bahasa Malaysia and Mandarin, too. Her teachers did not find her any different from her classmates. In fact, they commented on Mei's eloquence and intelligence.

Both girls were now in the same kindergarten—Mei in the older class, and Min Min in the younger. Min Min is now one of the most outgoing students in the little kindergarten. She enjoys school, has many friends, and is eager to learn. I did not disclose Min Min's developmental delay or her behavioral issues to the school, and her teachers never noticed anything different about her other than to remark that Min Min is very chatty in school.

A diagnosis of autism spectrum disorder needs to be revised, as evidenced by Mei's remarkable improvement in language and communication and marked reduction in stereotyped behaviors. June 2010

(Excerpt from Mei's psychological assessment)

In 2008, Mei scored 35.5 in the Childhood Autism Rating Scale (CARS), placing her within the moderate autism range. Only 1.5 points more and she would have been diagnosed with severe autism. Two years later, Mei scored 19.5 in the CARS rating, fully within the non-autistic range. We did other assessments, too, and all of them reported the same finding. Mei officially lost her autism diagnosis in exactly 2 years.

Mei graduated from kindergarten and is now in a mainstream private international school. Again, we chose not to disclose Mei's previous diagnosis, even though we have documented proof that Mei no longer has autism, not because I wanted to hide it from the school but because I didn't want her to be judged by it. Due to the preconceptions that come with an autism diagnosis, Mei had faced discrimination in the past. In her second kindergarten, her teachers only saw Mei as a child with autism, choosing to focus on her deficits and delays rather than on her strengths and abilities.

Mei loves her new school and teachers and has already made many friends in class. She is enjoying all of her new lessons and is more than capable of keeping up with her schoolwork and her classmates. Previously a child with severe social impairments, Mei now makes friends easily and enjoys a full and happy life.

My husband and I have endured many hardships throughout this journey, but it was Mei who worked the hardest of all. She overcame every challenge that life threw at her. I am humbled by her strength and courage. At times, I am guilty of holding Mei back, for autism has left far deeper scars in her compared to her little sister. If you look closely, you may still see the signs. She is an amazing girl albeit a little quirky. Mei is smart and brave, but within that strength there is a vulnerability that makes me want to hold her in my arms forever and protect her from the big, bad world. It is an urge I fight every single day. In order for her to soar, I have to let go.

Mei's sensitivity, intuition, depth of emotion, and complexity make her this unique little person whom the world is lucky to have. Autism may have prevented her from showing her love, but I knew she loved me deeply. My faith in Mei was rewarded tenfold; she has the biggest heart I know. The depth of her emotions stirs me. Her affection is obvious, her capacity for love and forgiveness is enormous, and she shows us her love every single day now.

Min Min is still in her kindergarten. She longs to be in the same school as Mei, but she has to wait one more year. I see no echoes of autism in her at all. I believe her language, cognition, and abilities are as typical as those of any child in her class. Min Min has acquired the social skills and killer charm that will hold her in good stead as she grows older. Her bright personality and intelligence shine every single day. I like to think that Min Min saves her biggest hugs and kisses for me. I tell her how much I love her and what she means to me every single night without fail. Even during the darkest days when autism kept a tenacious hold on our lives, I would try to find one bright moment: something to cherish, some way I could praise my daughters to let them know how proud I am of them.

Though Mei and Min Min have now recovered from autism, there are still lingering health issues. They still have immune dysfunction, gastrointestinal disorders, low muscle tone, and failure to thrive, to mention just a few. These issues will give rise to bigger and more serious medical illnesses if left unchecked. Healing takes a long time, and I am constrained by geography, bureaucracy, finances, and personal conflict.

The girls are no longer on strict dietary restrictions; however, I still encourage them to eat a healthy diet. We have phased out many of their less essential biomedical supplements and are complementing their treatment with homeopathy. Biomed got us to recovery, and I am hopeful that homeopathy will fill in the gaps, getting us to a deeper level of healing. At the moment, I can't tell what are quirks and what are remnants of autism. I know there's still some fine-tuning needed, but I'll gladly accept the quirks and oddities if my girls get their health back.

In the first few months after Mei's diagnosis, my fears were turning me into an autism victim. When I discovered that, I swore my family would not be victims to autism. My soul was slowly being eaten up by anguish. If I left it unchecked, it would fester in me, growing bigger and bigger, until I was drifting in an ocean of hurt. I chose to let go of the sadness and anger. Happiness is a choice: I could wallow in my grief and despair; I could dissect everything I ever did wrong; I could place the blame on many things and other people. Or I could choose happiness and joy instead. Yes, it is hard to feel happy when dealing with autism, but I see joy every day. While many people may see autism as a great burden, I do not. Mei and Min Min are my pride and joy. It is a privilege to be their mother.

Though the war on autism is over, we still feel like we're living in a war-torn zone, fighting a dirty, drawn-out battle, even though both parties have called a truce. The clean-up job is taking longer than the actual war. The scars run deep, and it will take a long time for us to recover from the physical and emotional toll to rebuild this family. It will take even longer to recover financially, though our initial investment has multiplied tenfold in other ways. We kicked the enemy's ass and regained our country. We are no longer autism victims, we are autism survivors.

My friend Tex introduced me to a group of amazing parents at the AutismOne conference, whose warmth and generosity of spirit made me feel at home. I graciously accepted their invitation to join an online group that would become The Thinking Moms' Revolution. Since then, I have been embraced by the collective spirit that is TMR. They inspire, motivate, and support one another. Their awesome brilliance and intellect make me honored to be a Thinking Mom. Thinking Moms are not backseat drivers; they are extraordinary mothers (and father). They make the earth spin and the valleys rock with their persistence, resilience, and tenacity.

There are four houses in Mei's school. Like Hogwarts, the houses compete against each other in sports, extracurricular activities, and academics, and at the end of the year the house with the most points is awarded a trophy. Unlike Hogwarts, Mei's school randomly assigns the houses. Mei was assigned the Green Dragon house. Her PE shirt is green with a white fire-breathing dragon on the front. When Mei wore the shirt for the first time, Hubby remarked that he had always thought of me as a dragon slayer. It was the first I'd heard of this. After much prodding, he finally explained that he views autism as a metaphorical dragon, blasting fire, chaos, and destruction everywhere. Along our journey, he has seen me slaying dragons—putting out fires and restoring order every single day. Ironic really, given that I've always viewed him as my knight in shining armor.

Biomedical resources in Malaysia have improved tremendously since Mei was diagnosed with autism. There are now three biomedical doctors here. In 2009, I founded KL Biomed, the first biomedical support group in Malaysia. KL Biomed is a support network for families affected by autism and related disorders who are doing biomedical interventions and alternative treatments. I am also the group owner and moderator of the KL Biomed Health Forum at http://health.groups.yahoo.com/group/klbiomed/.

Now, our members include families not just from Malaysia but also from Singapore, Indonesia, the Phillipines, and other Asian countries, including the Middle East. As a result, more and more families are implementing biomedical intervention and seeking alternative healthcare treatments. I am proud to have contributed to our community. I strive to advocate for biomedical and alternative healthcare treatments for children affected by autism, and I hope to continue empowering other parents to seek effective treatments for their children.

I am blessed to have recovered my children, yet too many families I know are still living with autism. Thanks to the many organizations and parent movements that believe that autism is treatable, we have hope and motivation to keep advocating for our children's right to better healthcare, education, and a brighter future.

Do . . .

- Go through this journey with grace and dignity. A thank you goes a long way: a smile even further.
- Have faith. Recovering a child from autism is a marathon, not a sprint. It takes hard work, perseverance, and faith— lots and lots of faith.
- Choose serenity. Autism has and still leaves a deep scar in our lives. I can choose to endure it grudgingly, with intense hatred and grief in my heart, or I can choose to make the best of it, with inner peace, grace, and serenity.
- Take care of your physical, mental, and emotional health. Don't forget to nourish your soul.
- Expect this to be a journey full of challenges and pitfalls. But also expect pleasant surprises and wonderful progress.
- Treat your children with kindness and respect.
- Make time to nurture your relationship if you are married. You are not the only one grieving; your spouse is too.
- Hang on to your sense of humor. Along the way, you will lose it, but try to regain it. You will need it.
- Have patience and learn to forgive.
- Set realistic goals. Give yourself small challenges.
- Celebrate the victories, small or big. Mourn the losses, but pick yourself up and keep going to the next level.

Don't . . .

- Sweat the small stuff. Look at the big picture. Think big, aim high.
- Forget to pray. Pray for good things.
- Underestimate your special child; you might just be pleasantly surprised.
- Let anybody hold you or your child back.
- Forget those who have helped you along the way. Pay it forward in the hopes that you too can help the next autism family that comes your way.

MOUNTAIN MAMA'S RECOVERY MISSION

Three weeks before his third birthday, my son was diagnosed with autism. As the panel of experts delivered the news, my world went silent. I could see mouths moving, and I'm sure there were comforting words, but I couldn't hear them. It was as if someone had turned down the world's volume. Later that day his therapist, Brooke, reminded me that he was the same sweet, beautiful child that he had been this morning before the diagnosis. I watched him play with his favorite toy—a tray full of spinning gears—pressing the button over and over, again and again. I knew Brooke was right, and I loved him as much as I ever had—probably more—but something was different. In a split second and with one word, my child had changed before my eyes. What I saw before me now was not just a precocious three-year-old. He was a victim—and so was I.

The days that followed were dark. My husband and I coexisted in a black fog of heartbreak. We didn't know what to say—nor what to do. We were simultaneously in overdrive to learn as much as we could and frozen in an emotional time warp. The earth kept spinning, but our world had stopped.

The following week would take us across the country to my brother's wedding. I had been looking forward to this trip for over a year, and now I was even more desperate to see family. I needed joy, celebration, smiles, hugs—or so I thought. What I really needed was to break down.

I had the whole trip planned perfectly. My boys were about to turn three and one. I had bought matching outfits for every event, including beautiful little beige linen suits. I was so proud of my little family, and I couldn't wait to show them off. I fantasized about the compliments I was sure to receive: "Oh, my God—look at your babies. They are *so* beautiful. And well-behaved. What a wonderful mother you are." Somehow in my zombie-like state of grief, I managed to get everything packed: favorite toys, special foods, diapers, cups, snacks for the plane, DVDs, cameras, strollers. Like all families with toddlers, we didn't travel light.

We didn't talk about it much, but Robert and I were nervous about how this would go. Traveling with small children is hard—throw autism in the mix, and it can be downright disastrous. We had to be out of the house at 5:00 a.m. to make our flight. The airport is an hour and a half from home, so the kids were done before we even started. Baker was mostly nonverbal then. He could answer the occasional question with echolalia: "Do you want some more juice?" "More juice." His eye contact was all but gone. It was beginning to return since we had started the diet and were killing yeast, but it was still bad—especially with strangers. He was easily overwhelmed and didn't handle chaos well. Transitioning from place to place might or might not bring a complete meltdown. He seemed to operate predominantly from a place of fear. The only thing predictable about my child was that he was unpredictable.

I thought I had anticipated everything that could have been a problem. I had played out from start to finish each step of the journey from parking and getting kids into strollers to going through security to getting on the plane, popping ears, take-off noises, confinement, changing diapers in that tiny bathroom, locating elevators and steering clear of escalators, keeping track of kids in crowds—you name it, I had mentally prepared myself for it all—except the looks.

I was firmly established in my role as victim, and unfortunately I wasn't quiet about it. I'll never know how many of the looks, stares, and comments throughout that trip were real and how many were imagined. I was certain that everyone was staring at us, wondering what was wrong with my child, thinking that we were horrible parents with an unruly, spoiled toddler. No one was safe from my irrational scrutiny. The poor cashier at McDonald's who told me they were out of straws was assaulted with "*What*? Out of straws? My child can't drink without a straw. He has autism. *Autism*. What the *fuck* are we supposed to do now?" The grandma that was simply trying to engage my three-year-old: "Hi. What's your name? I said, 'What's your name?'" "Sorry," I said. "He's shy. His name is Baker." "Oh. What a lovely name. Hi, Baker. How old are you? I said, 'How old are you?'" "He's three." "Oh, my grandson is four. He loves baseball. Baker, do you like baseball?" "*No*. He doesn't like baseball. He can't throw a ball, catch a ball, or say the word *ball*. He has *fucking* autism. Will you please leave us alone now?"

Despite my bad attitude and a few sensory overload meltdowns, we made it to Providence, rented a car, and drove to the beautiful house my brother had rented for my family. We were welcomed with warm smiles and long hugs by my parents. Baker did great. He gave hugs and kisses, accepted gifts gratefully and with delight. He let his Nana hold his hand and take him for walks. People were already there setting up for the rehearsal dinner being held in the lawn that evening. Relatives began trickling in one by one. I am very proud to be part of a large, loud, Irish Catholic family that lives for weddings and babies, and I was happy to provide the latter. I had been looking forward to this gathering for at least a year, but all of a sudden I felt sad and vulnerable. I didn't want to hear anything good about anyone. I just couldn't be happy for anyone who was still part of the world that had continued turning without us. No one seemed to see what I was so upset about. We had started the GFCF diet a couple of months ago, and even I had to admit that besides not talking, my child was acting more and more like a typical child. Throughout the night, he was happy, he danced, he allowed himself to be passed around from one relative to the next. As it was getting close to bedtime, Robert brought him in the bedroom where I was nursing the baby, lovingly surrounded by my aunts. I could tell by the horrified look on my husband's face that there was a problem. "I found him with a bag of hot dog buns. There are only three left." My heart sank into my stomach. My aunts laughed it off, "Isn't it cute—he got caught with his hand in the cookie jar." Robert and I were ready to cry.

The next morning, our beautiful, sweet toddler who had charmed an entire party had completely vanished. The person who had taken his place was new even to us. Baker had left. We couldn't reach him. He was terrified and had no idea what was happening, where he was, or what he was doing from one minute to the next. It was exactly like watching someone high on drugs. Those hot dog buns were the brown acid, and we had to stand by and watch our baby unravel.

The damage was done, and there wasn't anything we could do about it. We strapped him in the car seat and drove. We took him to an aquarium and tried to keep up as he ran from place to place, not able to stay in one place long enough to actually see much of anything. My family witnessed this whole episode and couldn't believe that he was the same child they had met the night before. I could see the confusion and pity on their faces. While their reaction made me sad, it also made me realize that we weren't crazy. Something as simple as a hot dog bun could turn my child's world upside down. I knew that we just had to make it through the next two days and then I would pull it together and do whatever I could to heal my child.

The next day I put on my new dress, dressed my boys in their suits, and looked proudly at my husband, who at that moment had transformed into the most handsome man I had ever seen. There is something about a father with sons in tow, all in their Sunday best that screams "family" to me. I knew how blessed I was to have him. I also knew that there was no way a few suits would hide the tragedy that was our life.

Once we got to the church, it became clear that Baker was not going to be able to make it through a quiet ceremony. My husband made the very selfless decision that I would not miss my brother's wedding. He would drive the kids around and meet me in the parking lot in an hour. I cried through the entire ceremony—I cried tears of joy for my brother, so happy that he had met the perfect complement to his beautiful spirit. I also cried because I had flash-backs of my own wedding, of all our hopes and dreams that had just been splattered like roadkill on our road to happiness.

Baker fell asleep in the car on the way to the reception. Robert and I took turns staying with him in the car and enjoying the party. My new sister-in-law had worked all year planning this reception—an incredibly elegant affair at a winery in Connecticut. It was per-fect. We didn't fit in this picture. There was no way I could enjoy this night—my heart was much too broken to celebrate anything. When Baker woke up, we considered taking him in the tent to eat and join the party. All I could think about was the cake and the tantrum that was sure to ensue as we tried to keep him away from it. We decided to leave and try to have some quiet time alone with him before bedtime. We watched him spiral and spin in his own world and eventually got him to sleep.

I waited up until my parents got home and pulled my mother aside. I had been waiting to be alone with her so I could fall apart. My mom held me as I literally crumbled to the floor. All I could say was "*Why?* Why did this happen? Why did this happen to my baby? What did I do wrong? Is God mad at me? *Why,* Mommy, *why?*" She held me as I sobbed and then picked me up off the floor and put me on the couch. She held my face in her hands, looked straight into my heart, and saw the pain that only another mother can see. Then she said, "My love, you are asking the wrong ques-tion. If Baker were healthy, would you ask, 'Why did God give me a healthy child?' Of course you wouldn't, so you don't get to ask 'Why?' now. God had nothing to do with this, and you know it. What you should be asking is 'How? How did this happen, and how are we going to fix it? How are we going to help him?' Those are the questions you need to ask." I stopped crying and looked at my mother, who had apparently turned into some kind of sage when I wasn't paying attention, and I could see in her eyes that she wasn't worried. Her heart was broken for me, but she wasn't worried. Somehow, that made me feel better, like she knew something that

I didn't and that everything would someday be okay. And I knew she was right. I didn't have the luxury of dwelling long in the Neverland of "Why?" I had to get on with "How?" I crashed hard that night and actually slept better than I had in months. Which was a good thing because the next two days were hell.

The next morning we packed, said our good-byes, and made our way to the airport. We turned in the rental car, and the nightmare began. We dragged our bags, our kids, and our already exhausted asses through ticketing and horrible security lines. Then we found our gate and set up base camp. The flight had been delayed, so we had two hours to kill. We let the kids run, we played on the moving sidewalks, we bought snacks, sodas, more snacks. We bought toys and books from the gift shop. Then the flight was delayed for two more hours. At this point, the kids were getting antsy. I was sure that the next two hours would go down as the longest two hours of my life. We were nervous and doing everything we knew to do to entertain a one-year-old and a three-year-old with autism. The meltdowns *were* coming; there was no way out of it if we had to stay there any longer. More than anything, we were physically exhausted. We had been carrying thirty-pound backpacks around for five hours while we chased the kids. We were done. We tried every possible escape route. Where was the closest airport? Could we rent a car and get there before the next flight left? What if we flew to a different airport, could we get a connection home? *Please get us out of here!* At that point I was playing the "A" card with the airlines—it didn't matter. We were stuck. And then they cancelled the flight. At this point, we were almost relieved. We just needed a bar and a bed, so a hotel sounded good.

We gathered our things, grabbed the shuttle, and got the kids set up in the room. Robert got us a six-pack, and we tried to calm down and make a plan. The next flight home wasn't until 5:00 p.m. the next day. We were stuck there—no food, no car, and no hotel after 11:00 a.m. We found flyers for the local zoo, got a bus schedule, and somehow managed to get the kids to sleep. Baker was at a place where bedtime rituals and routines were crucial. Being tossed from place to place was taking its toll, and we were witnessing the effects. We were doing the best we could with his diet, but it was becoming increasingly difficult.

The next day we packed up, hauled the kids to the bus stop, and made our way to the zoo. I was in the state of constant anticipation in which all autism moms reside, but otherwise things were going surprisingly well. We were actually having fun. We felt like a family—a damaged, frightened, imperfect one, but a family nonetheless. Then I noticed all the other families—their kids could talk about the animals, interact with their siblings, engage with their peers. I wanted what they had. I was beyond sad; I was *pissed*! How dare they parade around in all of their happiness and normalcy?! Didn't they know how much pain they were causing by their mere existence? I wanted to yell, scream, and knock the ice-cream cones out of their children's perfect little hands. Rational? No. But I couldn't help it. I wanted their life, the life I was *meant* to have, damn it! I wanted a relationship with my son. I didn't just want a functional family, I wanted a happy one, and I was determined to get it. I promised myself that day that I would do whatever it would take; I wouldn't stop until my son had recovered. It would be almost two years before I could stop comparing my son to typical kids and seeing only deficiency, comparing my family to theirs and seeing only shattered dreams.

The day after we got home, I found a DAN! doctor, did all appropriate medical testing, got started on an intense supplement routine, and enrolled Baker in a fabulous preschool. We paid for his teacher to go to a three-day workshop on teaching children with autism. We drove an hour each way three times a week in Montana winters for Baker to go to school and therapy. He responded well to all of our interventions. He began sleeping through the night. He started to potty train. He was rapidly rejoining our world, and while communication was a struggle and came slowly, he was a happy little boy. We became experts on what was going on with him internally. Running and crashing into things, laughing hysterically and inappropriately meant yeast. Loss of eye contact and increased stimming—food infractions. Tantrums, OCD, and rage—bacteria. We watched as his autism got better, but his health continued to decline. The more I learned about vaccines, the more I became convinced that my son's health issues were directly related. I learned that all vaccines could trigger an encephalitic reaction. The brain damage caused by encephalitis can present itself in different ways, including autism, seizure disorders, and immune diseases.

We were invited in the spring of 2010, when Baker was four and a half, to take part in a national study being conducted by Easter Seals and National Institute of Mental Health to explore the benefits of Floortime therapy. There were two groups, a control group that was not receiving any therapy services and an experimental group that received Floortime therapy training. We were part of the control group. What we would receive from taking part in the study was more testing and another autism screening by one of the nation's top professionals at administering the ADOS assessment. They would perform the assessments at the beginning of the study, when he was four and a half, and then again at the end of the study, when he would be five and a half. Because this was an independent study, I would not be obligated to share it with the school system, which meant I could have the testing done without running the risk of Baker losing services at school. It had been a year and a half since his initial ADOS screening and diagnosis. I was anxious but convinced that we had come so far that his place on the spectrum would be much higher.

For those unfamiliar with the ADOS, it works something like this. The scores fall between 0 and 24, where 0–7 means not on the spectrum, 8–12 is Asperger's, PDD, and high-functioning autism (HFA), anything over 12 is considered full-blown autism. The higher the number, the more severely impaired the child. Baker scored a 14 on his initial evaluation, and I was fully expecting that number to have fallen considerably. I was wrong. My heart sank into my stomach as I saw the exact same 14 staring back at me from the pages of the latest assessment. We had worked so hard; he had come so far. How could this be? How could he still be a 14? This would not do. I wiped the tears off of my face, put on my Google goggles, and started making phone calls.

I had been in almost daily contact with Blaze, a friend who had been on the biomed path with her son for years before we got started. She was—and is—my hero, and I credit her more than anyone else for how far my son has come. She told me that a lot of moms were trying homeopathy with their kids with good results. I felt like we had hit a wall with our recovery and knew it was time to try something different.

In the fall of 2010, Baker started kindergarten in an integrated classroom with a dedicated aide. He started homeopathy the same week. We dropped all interventions besides the diet and MB12 injections. He had been having terrible gut pain and had been referred to a GI specialist. We delayed the appointment and told ourselves we would give homeopathy three months to see improvement. Almost immediately we saw more language, cognitive improvement, and no more tummy pain. He had complained of tummy pain daily, and all of a sudden it was just gone. We realized that a dedicated aide was unnecessary. He was doing so much better than anyone had anticipated. The aide would remain in the classroom but only for support as needed.

The one drawback of healing was the new awareness about his social inadequacies. He longed for a friend and cried about the playground. I listened to my child cry and say the words, "I don't know how to play like those kids. There's something wrong with my brain. My brain is crazy, Mom. Why am I different?" I wasn't prepared for this, and I had no idea how to comfort him. Truth be known, I still don't.

We made it through kindergarten despite the social heartbreak and had the spring placement meeting. Robert and I had assumed that, due to his social struggles and the fact that he had missed so much school due to illness, he would have to repeat kindergarten. Our big concern on the way to the meeting was how to explain to him that he would be repeating kindergarten without damaging his self-esteem. We were informed that under no circumstances would Baker be recommended for retention. He was performing in the average range right alongside his classmates. He would need to be in a classroom with an aide for redirection, help with focusing, and occasional one-to-one help due to fine-motor and processing problems. I knew that we had made progress, but this conversation surpassed all of my hopes. He was doing it. He was going to be OK.

Later that week, we filed in the auditorium with all of the other parents to watch our children "graduate" from kindergarten. We watched as they said the alphabet, sang the days of the week, and twirled on stage pridefully counting by fives and tens. I watched my son struggle to keep up, and oddly twitch and spasm. These new jerky, odd movements had been concerning me for a while. The stage lights were bright and blaring. I watched helplessly as Baker stared into the blood-red glowing cylinder and began to contort. I grabbed Robert's hand. I watched ready to jump up and grab him. What was happening? His whole body began to fold in on itself, and it was obvious he wasn't in control. It lasted about ten seconds, and then he began to jump up and down and rejoined the song. I was sobbing uncontrollably. Everyone around me thought I was emotional because of the occasion. I knew I had just witnessed my son having a seizure and was terrified. Luckily, the performance had been filmed, and I was able to hand it over to the neurologist who confirmed that my son had in fact had a complex-partial seizure. He handed us our prescription for anticonvulsants and sent us on our way.

Two weeks passed, and I received the results of the final ADOS screening for the Easter Seals study. I remembered proudly how well my son had performed that day. I had felt the exact same way the first two times we had been through this screening. I had prepared myself for the worst and told myself that it didn't matter. It was just a stupid number, and one assessment couldn't take into account all of our successes. No matter how bad it was, I would stay positive and focus on progress and my son's beautiful spirit. I sat in the car at the post office with the kids in the back seat. I ripped the envelope carelessly and with an apathetic attitude, skipped the formal letter and explanation of diagnostics, and scanned the pages for that stupid number. There it was: Total Communication and Social Interaction Score: 4. "Your child's Total Communication and Social Interaction Score indicates that at pre-test, your child met the criteria for autism. At post-test, your child met the criteria for No Dx." I sat in the car and read those words over and over. "No Dx." Then I began to laugh—like a crazy woman. The kids started laughing with me. I was crying now too. "What's funny, Mommy? Tell us the joke. Did you read a funny joke?" "Yes, my love. But the joke's on them, and we got the last laugh." I drove straight to my husband's jobsite and crashed into the poor man in hysterics. I told him the news and watched him *not* react. "What the hell is wrong with you? I just told you that your son lost his diagnosis. Didn't you hear me?" He looked at Baker smiling and waving in the back seat of the car. "I heard you," he said, "and I'm happy, but it doesn't really change anything, does it? He's still really behind. He is still really sick. This doesn't mean that it's over." But something had changed. With one number, my son went from being a victim to a child full of potential. In an instant, I stopped comparing him to other children and seeing deficiencies. Now I saw him only as himself, a child on his own developmental path.

When my husband came home, I could tell by his smile that he had been thinking and processing the news. He was ready to celebrate with me. We took turns playing devil's advocate and listing all of the reasons this couldn't be real. What we ultimately decided to do would be an experiment. We would go on a minivacation to celebrate. We booked a room at a little hotel with hot springs mineral pools that smelled strongly of sulphur. The hotel was having a music festival, so there would be loud music and chaotic crowds. The rooms had no air conditioning or television. This would take Baker out of his routine, out of his comfort zone, and throw him into a sensory nightmare. We knew that a child in the throes of autism would never be able to handle this trip.

We made the two-hour trip in only three and a half hours and fewer than fifty "Are we there yet?" There was loud music on the lawn, people dancing, and celebration in the air. We fit right in. Baker's response three years ago would have been to clasp his hands over his ears and scream in panic at the sound. His reaction today was: "Look, Mom—a band! When I grow up, I'm going to play the tuba. Look, people are dancing. I can dance. Do you like my dancing, Mom? Check out these moves."

We put on our swimsuits and headed down to the mineral pools. They smelled just like boiled eggs. Three years ago, we would have had screaming and crying over the smell. I would have panicked and fled. Today, he said, "Yuck. It smells like eggs. I hate eggs. Come on, Mom. Watch me do a cannonball."

Okay. So we have the sensory overload beat, but what about the chaos and the people? There are a lot of kids in this pool. "Mom, that boy took my kickboard. He can play with it, but will he keep it forever?" "Of course not," I said. "I think it is really nice that you're letting him use your kickboard. When you want it back, just go tell him that it's yours and you would like it back." "But, Mom, I don't know his name." "Well, then I guess you'll have to ask him." I watched as he waded over to the other child and asked much too quietly for the child to hear "What's your name?" and again "What's your name?" Finally, he yelled "*I said, 'What's your name?'*" A couple on the edge of the pool had been watching him and began to laugh. I laughed, too, and made some comment about how we are still working on our social skills. The man shook his head and said, "No, I think it's great. He's great." His wife agreed and added, "Look how social he is . . . Look at him trying to make friends." With that comment, I knew we had done it. We still had a long way to go, but this was *not autism*. Not anymore.

I wanted to scream it from the rooftops, put up a billboard, go on television—I wanted to show the world that autism is treatable. My son had autism, and now he doesn't. I had always been up front about Baker's autism. I was heartbroken by it but never ashamed of it. I would never give it that power. Having said that, I never would have made my child the poster child for autism. But the poster child for recovery—sign us up. Then it occurred to me. Recovery. Recovery. We weren't there. Nowhere close. At the same time I was celebrating the fact that we had sent autism packing, I was monitoring my son's visual field for seizure triggers. "Baker, stop staring at that sprinkler." "Baker, quit looking at that neon light." "Yes, babe. The moon is beautiful—quit looking at it."

The tics and seizure activity had been more and more frequent. He couldn't go anywhere with fluorescent lights, which was making daily life logistically difficult.

So this is where we are. I find myself in the very awkward position of having a child who lost his diagnosis but is a long way from recovered. I have had a hard time reconciling these facts. As I have worked and prayed and researched and grieved, I somehow always thought that "no diagnosis" would look different. I thought it would at least *resemble* recovery. My child is still very much affected in so many ways. He struggles with conversational language and has global dyspraxia, dyslexia, and seizures. His immune system is compromised, and he seems to stay sick. His gross and fine motor skills are extremely delayed. He struggles socially, although everyone seems to like him. We are lucky that the teasing and bullying hasn't started yet, although I am already mentally preparing myself for that day. He still obsesses over toys and stims when he is sick or tired.

Because "lost diagnosis" does not equal "recovery," I have been very hesitant to tell our story. Because he is not 100 percent recovered, people have a hard time believing that he lost his diagnosis. Some people have even suggested that he must have been misdiagnosed initially and never *really* had autism. Some people have suggested that he must have just really had a good day when he had his last assessment. I would like to put these two theories to rest. My son was diagnosed two years in a row by two different child psychologists and received the exact same score. Three years after his initial diagnosis, he did not meet the criteria for a diagnosis. A child with autism can't test out of a diagnosis—even on the best day. I am very proud of how far we have come and how hard he worked to get here. To deny his diagnosis is to deny his pain and his work.

Other people have shared in our happiness and celebrated this news with an understanding that our life is still imperfect. Throughout this journey, I have had the pleasure of meeting some of the smartest, kindest, dedicated, and compassionate women on the planet. They have helped me put together this puzzle, piece by piece.

I have cried when their children have been in pain, and celebrated when they made progress. Every new word, every day of potty training, every sleepless night, fever, trip to the doctor, every failed play date—we are there for each other. Unfortunately, because our relationships have developed over the phone and Internet, I have never been able to thank these women properly for their friendship. They have been there for me in ways that people in my real community never could be.

I live in a very small town. My son is one of only two children with autism in our community. This has felt very isolating at times. We just didn't fit in this community, so I found a different one. My community spans from Hong Kong to Montreal, from Malaysia to Texas. I belong to a community of fighters. We fight schools, doctors, insurance companies, illnesses, and the misconceptions of autism. We fight our own demons, our feelings of despair. We fight for the courage and the energy to go on. We exist in a different realm. We left the shiny, glimmering surface of normal life with clean houses, new clothes, and coffee talk for the deep, dark depths of autism. In some ways, I have allowed my son's autism to define not only him but me as well. I am an autism mom—and I couldn't be prouder. When Baker lost his diagnosis, I no longer knew exactly where I fit. Am I still an autism mom? Without autism, who was I? Technically speaking, autism could be out of our life. I could make my way back to the surface and move on, but the truth is that I can never go back. Not while children and families are still hurting. As long as autism is part of this world, I am a part of the world of autism.

Believe it or not, there *are* gifts that come along with autism. I am a better mother because of my son's diagnosis. I read and understand food labels, clean my house with vinegar instead of toxic cleaners, grow organic food, use nontoxic cookware, and treat illnesses as naturally as possible. I am a better person because of autism. I can use words like "resilient," "patient," "compassionate," and "nonjudgmental" to describe myself now. Those are not the words that would have described me prior to autism. When my children learn new skills or have successes, I don't take it for granted. My heart feels joy in a way that mothers of neurotypical children will never experience.

Our life is far from perfect. My son has not recovered; I have not recovered, but we are healing. We are a family in every sense of the word, and not just a functioning family but a happy one. My son is on a soccer team with his brother and neurotypical kids. He is in cub scouts. He is finding his way in a world that will hopefully one day embrace him and his beautiful, kind, fragile spirit. There are still bad days and failed attempts, but we have more good days than bad, more successes than failures. We still get "the look" from strangers from time to time, but I no longer feel compelled to justify my son's differences with the autism explanation. Let them wonder. I will continue to fight for full recovery for my son, and I believe with all of my being that we will get there. My son asked me what I was writing. I told him that I was writing a story about us. "Does it start with 'Once upon a time? Stories are supposed to start with 'Once upon a time.'"

"No, my love. Not this story. But I promise it will end with 'happily ever after.'"

SUGAH'S SPICY TALE

Lying on the living room floor with my feet propped up on the sofa, I could feel my blood coursing through my veins. My body ached intensely, just like it did after my last six-mile hike. I was starting to get concerned because I had given my body three days of rest between hikes. I thought back to just six months ago, before we moved to Alaska. Back then, I loved to go for long speed walks in the spring and fall, but I would retreat to the comfort of my temperature-controlled home and my elliptical machine during the sweltering 100-degree and 99 percent humidity days of southeast Texas. Back then, I would stay on that machine for an hour and a half, getting off only because I had other things to do. I would work out twice a day many times. I loved it.

But here I was, lying on the floor with my aching body. At times, the muscle pain was unbearable. My health had taken a downward turn since we moved to the cold northern-Alaskan climate just six short months before: fatigue, foggy thinking, absence of stamina, hormonal fluctuations, irritability. The list went on. I tried to wrap my brain around it. Friends would ask me if I was homesick. I mean, I *loved* living in Texas, but I was very excited about moving to Alaska. Adventure! I moved there with aspirations of training for adventure racing. We even bought a house two blocks away from a sixteen-mile hike/bike trail. I had big plans! But within six months, my whole world had turned upside down.

I would eventually learn that people with mercury poisoning do not fare well in extreme temperatures. There is a subset of people who have a difficult time dealing with the change in climate that occurs during the fall and winter months. Some people call it SAD, seasonal affective disorder. Many of those suffering with SAD have undiagnosed mercury poisoning. My mercury poisoning was a direct result of childhood cavities that were filled with amalgam—"silver"—fillings.

In addition to the angst I felt for my own declining health condition, concerning reports were coming home from school. My older son had been acting strangely. He wouldn't do the same pre-school "work" that his peers were doing. There was little interaction with the other children. He didn't answer questions appropriately or look you in the eye. He would do this galloping movement around the room. I knew this meant something. I couldn't ignore it. I had to dig in and research what the teacher was telling me. Online, I discovered the concept of nonverbal learning disorder. It sounded so much like my son's condition.

My husband and I had been concerned off and on about our older son. We would talk about things that we saw that were concerning. Then my husband would read an article about autism on CNN.com or another news outlet. We would take comfort in the fact that our son did not have the same symptoms described in those articles. This concern-read-denial cycle happened several times.

Once, I took him to our pediatrician in Texas and talked with her about our concerns. She gave me a reassuring pat on the back and told me there was nothing to worry about; he would grow out of it. I really wanted to believe her. And I did . . . for a while.

Since he was our first child, we didn't have anyone else to compare him to. My mother-in-law kept telling me how he was developing exactly like my husband did. I would take comfort in those words and brush off my fears. I was living in denial.

Not long after the excruciating six-mile hike, I took my older son to the doctor's office for his fifth-birthday checkup. I had diligently taken my children to the doctor for every well-child checkup.

I made sure they received all their vaccinations on time because I wanted my children to have the best chance for a healthy life. The doctor walked into the room. There were large stickers of cars up on the walls. My son wanted to touch them. He climbed up on the exam table to touch the stickers on that wall, but he couldn't reach the ones on the other walls. The doctor, who had been watching his every move, walked over and picked him up. He carried my son to the other walls so that he could touch every sticker in the room. After my son was finished, I saw the look of satisfaction on his face. The doctor looked at me and said something like, "The autism spectrum is rather big, and there are many different kinds of children on it." He knew right away.

Denial was no longer a possibility.

I quickly scheduled the first available appointment with a child psychologist, who eventually diagnosed my son with mildly moderate autism. I remember clearly asking her, "What can I do to fix this? I'll do anything!" She looked me straight in the eye and explained that autism is an incurable neurological disease. There was nothing but standard therapy that could be done for him. He would always have autism.

My biggest accomplishments in life have followed instances in which somebody has told me I couldn't do something.

I didn't know it at the time, but this was a life-changing moment for my family. Nothing else would ever be the same. I would no longer live my life as someone who blindly listened to those in authority when it came to the well-being of my children. I would now and forever question everything I heard, and trust only those who did the same.

Of course, this change in me didn't happen overnight. It took many months. The psychologist's words burned in my ears. She was a professional. She spent a long time in school and had lots of letters that followed her name. It was hard for me to fathom that what she told me could be completely wrong. But I had an itch, a feeling of uneasiness that I wasn't supposed to just sit there and accept this diagnosis. I knew I had to question it, but I had no idea where to start. So I turned on my computer.

Surfing the web one day, I ran into tacanow.org. It was so help-ful and so overwhelming at the same time. The list of things to do to help one's child recover was so long. And I still had the psychol-ogist's antagonistic voice in my head telling me to give it up. After a few hours of reading, the words were flying around my head in a tornado of stress. I didn't know whom to trust. Didn't know whom to listen to. The psychologist, with many years of formal education and lots of letters behind her name, or tacanow.org.

I decided to give it a month. I decided to try the gluten-free, casein-free diet for a month. I told myself, "If there are any changes at all, then I'll take this recovery thing seriously."

It only took eleven days. The first ten days were hell, but the eleventh day was a day of awakening. On the way to preschool, my son said, "Mom, look at that tree. There are *leaves* on it!" We were driving the same route we had taken to preschool every day for many months, but it was like he was looking at it all for the very first time.

We were so full of hope with our older son's startling improve-ment on the gluten-free, casein-free diet. At the same time, my con-dition seemed to be getting worse. I went to see a doctor and told him my symptoms: debilitating fatigue, irritability, lack of stamina, muscle aches, and intense brain fog, amongst others. He offered to put me on an antidepressant. I was astonished! I wanted to say, "Seriously? Is that the best you've got?" I was *sick*. I might have been sad that I was sick, but I was definitely sick before I became sad. I said, "No, thanks!"

Given my recent experience with the child psychologist, I had already begun to question the authority of the medical establishment. However, the experience of being offered antidepressants had per-manently changed how I looked at medical doctors. I understood now that my health, and the health of my family, was in my hands. So I began to research. I spent hours looking at various natural healing websites, searching for natural cures for autism and chronic fatigue. Then one day it hit me. The cures and lifestyle recommen-dations that I found for chronic fatigue were very similar—and in some cases exactly the same—as the recommendations that I found to heal my son from autism. I could sense that there was something bigger going on, but I couldn't quite put my finger on it.

There were many books that I read in the early days of this journey, but one book in particular changed my whole point of view and approach to healing my family: *Healing the New Childhood Epidemics*, by Kenneth Bock, MD. In this book, I learned about the causative factors for not only autism but most childhood diseases. Proliferation of chemicals and toxins in our environment and in our food supply, and the increase in childhood vaccinations combine to create a condition of metabolic dysfunction and cellular toxicity.

Now the dots were starting to connect. It was starting to make sense. All the Internet research I had done about my chronic fatigue and the research on autism overlapped and blended together. My illness and my son's illness had the same root cause: chemical and other exposures to toxins by way of our environment, food supply, vaccinations, and dangerous dental practices.

I started to think about my younger son. He had the EXACT same chemical and toxin exposures that his older brother had. Why didn't he have autism? There was not even a glimmer of autism in his behavior. He loved to engage people in conversation or silly banter to make them smile. Gregarious. Loving. But having pledged myself to never live in Denial Land again, I had to take a serious look at him. My younger son had the same childhood illnesses as his older brother: ear infections followed by tube surgery, croup, lots of antibiotic use. And while he seemed generally neurotypical, still there were a few things about him that were "off." I watched him in a therapist's waiting room. He *had* to touch *everything*. Compulsively. His teachers complained about his behavior and his inability to do the same preschool "work" that his peers were doing. He also was chronically constipated. Something was definitely not right.

Eventually, we would have tests run on both boys: tests to determine heavy metal loads, tests to determine viral, bacterial, and other pathogen loads. All of the tests showed that my neurotypical younger child was *more* toxic than my child with autism. Shocking.

What are we dealing with here?

In my one little family we have a mother—me—with chronic fatigue, one child with autism, and another child with ADD/impulsive/inattentive tendencies. Could this all be related? Why, yes, it was.

In time, I would learn and understand that the vast majority of mental, emotional, and physical issues that children and adults experience have the same root cause. The label given to the mental, emotional, and/or physical issue will be different based on the symptoms that an individual presents, but the root cause does not change. This includes autism, allergies, PTSD, anxiety, bipolar depression, ADHD, learning disabilities, food allergies, diabetes, asthma, Crohn's, lupus, chronic fatigue, fibromyalgia, MS, ME, arthritis, cancer, heart disease, seizure disorders, epilepsy, mitochondrial disorder, etc. In my opinion, regardless of the label, the underlying medical condition and root cause are the same: environmental toxins causing immune dysfunction, resulting in systemic inflammation, metabolic disorder, chronic cellular toxicity, and pathogen imbalance.

In order to really comprehend the concept of "all diseases—one root cause," we first have to understand what it means to be healthy and how we get sick.

What does it mean to be healthy?

When you eat, your body breaks down the food to be used or stored as energy. In proper metabolism, your body uses enzymes to complete a complex set of chemical reactions that function to maintain life, produce energy, and facilitate detoxification. In some of these chemical reactions, your body will break down and excrete substances that it no longer needs or create substances that it is lacking. So when you are healthy, and your body is working properly, you are able to detox—or get rid of—substances your body does not need, and you can create substances that your body does need.

What about when your body is not working properly?

When too many toxins enter your body, your organs for detoxification get overwhelmed. When your liver cannot process and remove all of the toxins, the toxins are left to circulate in your blood and lymph system. Toxins interfere with enzyme production, hormone regulation, and the normal course of chemical reactions that occur in a healthy metabolism. The lack of adequate enzymes results in the building of chemical imbalances and circulation of exogenous toxins. The excess chemicals and toxins cause systemic inflammation, which interferes with proper brain function. The toxins settle in tissues and eventually embed themselves within the cell walls, leading to a condition of chronic cellular toxicity. A dysfunctional liver and the absence of required enzymes lead to immune dysfunction. The body is unable to fight off offending bacteria, virus, fungus, parasites, and other pathogens furthering systemic inflammation. The body becomes acidic, and disease thrives. This state of systemic inflammation, disordered metabolism, chronic cellular toxicity, and pathogen imbalance manifests itself in a variety of different physical, mental, and behavioral challenges. The differences in the type of toxin in question, where/in what tissues it is embedded, and your genetic predisposition will determine which symptoms you will exhibit and, therefore, which diagnostic label you will receive. A child may be labeled with autism, Asperger's, ADD/ADHD, ODD, learning disability, asthma, allergies. An adult may be labeled with chronic fatigue, fibromyalgia, diabetes, cancer, PTSD, bipolar, depression. Older adults may carry the Parkinson's or Alzheimer's labels.

Back to my family. My poor health condition had its beginnings from childhood cavities filled with dental amalgam ("silver"). I might have been okay if we had just left them there. Maybe. Many people live their whole lives with amalgams and never seem to have any problems. But then again, many will develop diabetes, chronic fatigue, or other chronic illnesses that have their roots in metabolic disorders.

Ground zero of my health problems occurred during my preteen years, on the day I had my amalgams removed by a general dental practitioner who did not specialize in safe amalgam removal. You see, he just put his drill in my mouth and tiny particles of mercury embedded in my gums. And there began my mercury toxicity. It was the beginning of my immune dysfunction. Almost immediately, I began to contract regular acute illnesses like strep throat and bronchitis. As a teenager, I would observe that my internal thermometer was not working properly. I would notice that my skin was unusually cold and clammy when it should have been hot and sweaty while playing sports. Later in life, I developed anaphylactic food allergies. Looking back, I know that I also was suffering from candida overgrowth. When it came time to have children, I needed the assistance of a fertility specialist in order to ovulate. I was blind to so many red flags that are now, reflectively, so clear to me.

When my first child was born, I thought I was healthy. I worked out a lot and was in top physical shape. I was eating a pretty good diet. I was blind to the fact that my food allergies and my need of fertility assistance were key indicators of a radically dysfunctional immune system. My first child bore the brunt of my toxic burden. I have heard that a developing fetus chelates toxins away from the mother and into its own body and that that's one reason the first child is so often more affected than subsequent children.

There was no dramatic regression into autism with my first son. In my belly, he did not move around very much. He was already poisoned by the mercury in my body. His in utero mercury poisoning was further aided by a complete vaccine schedule. Looking back at his medical records, there is a clear pattern of vaccination followed by illness. I was blind to the connection at the time, but looking reflectively at his medical records, the association is clear. I confused his incredible ability to recite books and movies with real communication. So my first son was not diagnosed with autism until he was five.

Regardless of age or degree of functioning, there is always hope for functional improvement and possibly even recovery.

My oldest son will be nine this month and is very close to recovery. Some days it feels like we are really far away, but at other times it feels like recovery is in our midst. Either way, there is a light at the end of the tunnel. *Go big, or don't go at all.* Yes, that's one of my mantras. And just so you'll understand my expectations, I want my son to be indiscernible from his peers. I don't want just a little recovery; I want it all.

Organ support, detoxification, and brain retraining is our plan.

We have been working hard on recovery. We have tried many, many, many different protocols, therapies, and supplements in order to get where we are. The things that have worked really well for our family are Andy Cutler's chelation, homotoxicology, and classical homeopathy. There are many other things that we have done, but these are the protocols that provided us with the most detoxification.

Brain retraining is our new horizon. We are just about finished with detox—removing the toxins, metals, viruses, bacteria, and parasites from our bodies and brains. What's left will be the neurological pathways that didn't develop correctly during early childhood— those neurological pathways that were blocked very early on in life by toxins. Those brain connections may very well have to be rebuilt. The good news is that it has been proven possible. Neuroplasticity. This is our new focus. Our new challenge. Our new hope.

PRINCESS GIVES PRAISE

The story I am about to share with you details my family's journey over the past nine months. It is a beautiful story. Every part of it feels like it has been directly sent from G-d, with love and deliberateness.

At the beginning of this journey, my four-year-old, nonverbal son with autism was receiving thirty hours of verbal behavior therapy in one of the finest school districts in the country. He also received several hours of occupational, physical, and speech therapies there. We spent the entire school year advocating for the school to add more social instruction to his program and less ABA. Our son never responded positively to ABA. In fact, I would say he responded negatively. Prior to ABA, he was loving and trusting of us. Once we started ABA, he became a defiant, tantrum-prone, and miserable little guy. He was not only unable to express himself but he also became untrusting of everyone who tried to help him. When he recently changed those behaviors, we realized that we had created them in the first place.

All year, there were things about the school that had rubbed me the wrong way: the questions they asked out of obligation and formality without the slightest expression of emotion on any professional's face; the patronizing explanations they gave to us, his "ignoramus parents"; and most of all, the complete lack of expression of love for N. The teachers seemed to begrudgingly march the children around from point A to point B, waiting for each school day to end. Despite this gut feeling, I felt too desperate to pull him out of this school. I had no alternative that I knew of, and the idea of having him home all day to stim (self-stimulate) to his heart's content was unimaginable to me. So, I continued "fighting the fight" with blood, sweat, and tears in each IEP meeting. I walked away from those meetings with paltry services that didn't even allow me to pretend that I was doing the right thing for him.

I began researching. I started reading about the Son-Rise Program at the Autism Treatment Center of America (ATCA). I had heard about it a year earlier on a Yahoo! group. I read something about loving and accepting your child along with his stimming (or *ism*-ing as they call it), and I rolled my eyes thinking, "What apologetics; this must be the new fad—since we can't change autism, let's all pretend we love it and dance around a campfire singing 'Kumbaya.'" But when I saw their website for the first time, I got a totally a different vibe.

Founded by Barry Neil Kaufman and Samahria Lyte Kaufman, the Son-Rise Program was developed by a loving couple who refused to give up hope for their severely autistic son. After being told to institutionalize their son, who had an IQ of less than 30, they decided to join him in his world instead. Whereas conventional and mainstream therapies try to stop or prevent a child from engaging in repetitious behaviors, the Son-Rise Program encourages the parents to join their child in these actions. By doing so, one creates a more loving and trusting relationship, which then allows the child to feel safe enough to join our world. Today, their son, Raun, is the CEO of the Option Institute and Autism Treatment Center of America, an international lecturer, teacher, and group facilitator with a near-genius IQ and not a single trace of autism. (For more information about the Son-Rise Program, visit www.autismtreatment.org.)

After learning more about Son-Rise, I realized it was exactly what we were looking for. I recognized that I had completely misunderstood their philosophy. While you do fully accept your child, you are not simply settling and are not without goals for him, as I had previously thought. The Son-Rise Program has a very unique set of techniques and principles, which, when applied, can bring about full recovery from autism!

Shortly after my realization, the ultimate stroke of fate happened. Soon after registering for the AutismOne conference in Chicago, I received an informational email. I opened it as soon as it hit my inbox. It said that the first forty people to reply would receive a full week of free childcare by the professional Son-Rise staff! It sounded marvelous, and I replied right away. At the time, I didn't realize just how lucky we were to have this opportunity. In just those short few days, N started to open up. It was undeniable! The most beautiful part was the tremendous, palpable love and warmth the facilitators had for him. We didn't know the facilitators at all, yet we could feel their love every time we entered the room. One day, we walked in and saw N jumping in the middle of the room with his arms wrapped around another child's neck in an embrace, laughing! That was all it took; we were immediately sold. We started learning and implementing the Son-Rise techniques with him in the evenings. There was a glimmer of something amazing shining through.

On our drive back to Connecticut, we stopped at a gas station. We needed to let him out of the car to stretch his legs, but we weren't sure how to accomplish this because we knew he would run off. Ordinarily, we would spend our time chasing after him while yelling for him to come back to the car. This time was different. Inspired by our experience, we ran with him celebrating. To our amazement, for five straight minutes, he began to run back and forth between us, laughing and throwing himself into our open arms. My husband and I could not believe what we were seeing. Although we didn't know exactly what the Son-Rise Program entailed, we did know that we had to pursue it further. The staff had mentioned a Start-Up program in June or August that we could attend. We wanted to attend the one in June, but it was only a month away, and both of us were still students; we just didn't have the funds for it. We decided to try to attend the Start-Up program in August.

August seemed so far away. We received a call from ATCA to talk with one of their family counselors. He was extremely patient with us. He worked with us at our pace and tried to comfort all of our qualms. Despite many passing weeks during which we had done absolutely nothing to get ourselves to the program, our family counselor called us religiously to check on our progress. He planted a seed about fundraising the money we needed, an idea that previously would have been unfathomable to us.

We got back to our regular lives feeling passionate and infused. We told the school about Son-Rise and received their dutiful statement, "Oh, yes, we'd love to learn more about it." At that point, we felt like rogue parents. The more we learned about Son-Rise, the more we realized that our instincts about the school had been right all along. Their program was destructive for N. We wanted to run a Son-Rise Program for N, but we were at a loss of where to begin. We didn't know what to do, and we didn't have the money to get to the training.

One morning, I brought my sweet guy to school, and he bolted to the soccer fields. He always had a hard time with transitions in general, so arriving at school was always a challenge. But this morning was different. With my fifteen-month-old baby in tow, I raced after him and tried to maneuver him back to the sidewalk and toward the building. Once I'd managed to drag him up to the sidewalk, he threw a tantrum and flung himself down on the ground. I'd started reading about the idea of joining a child while he or she stims, and I didn't really understand exactly how to do it, but in this moment joining him seemed better than fighting him. So, with baby in hand, I laid down on the pavement next to him. Immediately, I got panic-stricken stares from other parents. Soon after, his teacher ran out from about twenty feet away and dragged him into the classroom. I felt so much heartache in that moment. I didn't want to force him to go to school, but I was desperate and without the proper tools to have him at home.

That day—which happened to be a Friday—at about five o'clock in the afternoon, I got a phone call from the school's special ed director telling me that N was physically abused by one of his paraprofessionals. When I asked who she was, the director refused to tell me. At that moment, it was clear to me that he would not be going back to that school ever again, no matter what.

The several weeks that followed felt distressing. We had no program or infrastructure for him at home, but we couldn't send him back to school. After weeks of investigating with the Department of Children and Families (DCF), we learned more about what had transpired. Apparently, another paraprofessional reported to DCF that she witnessed N sitting on a beanbag with another child. N started to get aggressive, or was about to get aggressive, when the paraprofessional, a fill-in for lunchtime and whose name I'd never heard before, flung him down, causing him to smack into a chair before hitting the floor. The school's attempt to cover up this whole event was especially concerning. They sent him to the nurse to be examined that day and noticed that his back had a red bruise. They sent him home and allowed us to send him back the next day, without mentioning anything. This is the very same nurse, by the way, who never hesitated to send him home many times for diarrhea. Yet now that a teacher had physically abused him, neither the nurse nor anyone else thought it was necessary to call home. The next day, they sent him back to the nurse for a reexamination. Again with no phone call home. Finally, at five o'clock the day after the incident, we received a reluctant call from the school. We later discovered that the call only came because they'd realized that one of their paraprofessionals had already reported the incident.

Because we did not know about the incident, we brought N to school the day after it happened. That was the morning that he bolted for the soccer fields. Suddenly, I understood why he ran! He was trying to tell me that he didn't want to go to school and that he wasn't safe there. I had written his behavior off as autism, rather than an important attempt at communication, and allowed him to be dragged through the school's doors. Now, after being trained in Son-Rise, I know that I will never ignore another attempt at communication again. Although our children might not have all the tools necessary to communicate with us, they are extremely intelligent beings, who should not be disregarded. In fact, when I really thought about it, he had resisted getting out of the car every morning. Now I wonder if they had been rough with him all year.

We scurried about for a while considering our options: Go to court and fight the school? Send him to a private school? The more we dissected each of these options, the more we realized we just didn't have the money for any of them. Furthermore, with both of us being full-time graduate students, we had no flexibility in our schedules. We could spend a fortune paying a lawyer's retainer fee, with no guarantee that we would be successful (and what did we even want from the school anyway?), or we could spend the money making an actual program that would help him.

Other than to validate my original instincts that the school was a destructive setting for N, the details of this story really aren't important to me anymore. I'm incredibly grateful that all this happened. I see it as a blessing because it was this drastic event that finally forced me to do what I should have done long before. That fateful Friday marked N's last day in school. The summer was long and difficult. Still lacking the structure and training necessary to run our own Son-Rise Program, we frantically tried to get through each day, with an iPad and TV as our regrettable babysitters. We spent this challenging transitional period wholeheartedly loving our son, and he could feel it. He was happy to be home, and we were excited at the prospect of our future Son-Rise Program.

After many long talks with our incredibly calm and patient family counselor at the Option Institute, we decided to fundraise to get ourselves to the Son-Rise start-up training in August. We sent out a mass email to our closest friends and family, detailing the program and our experience with it in Chicago. We were met with some small donations and letters of support, along with some more adversarial emails that recommended exactly what treatment those individuals believed we should be pursuing. We heard rumors from family that some thought our hopes and dreams of Son-Rise, as well as our fundraising efforts, were inappropriate and unrealistic. At the time, this really hurt, but several months later, I realized that it forced us to stand by our choice and become what the Option Institute refers to as a "force of nature." We chose to make attending the start-up training our purpose, and we had conviction. We took daring action by standing up to opposition. We felt passionate about our choice and persisted until we made it a reality. I personally believe that because we did that, G-d stepped in and helped us the rest of the way.

In just a short while, we had raised enough money to make our way to the start-up program. This five-day program taught us all about joining our son in his repetitive behaviors as a way of interesting him in us and our world. We learned about loving and accepting him fully while striving for him to grow without needing him to. We learned about how to celebrate even his smallest efforts at communicating with energy, excitement, and enthusiasm. We learned about how to set up our special distraction-free playroom. We learned how to recruit and train volunteers. We learned how to love ourselves better. We made great friends. And we left feeling empowered and excited.

Since returning home, things have moved at an unstoppable pace. In the past few months, we've set up our playroom, received enough in donations to help us fund our program this year, and recruited twelve volunteers to come to our home to work with our son in two-hour shifts from morning to evening, seven days a week. I've since been back to the ATCA for two incredible, life-changing advanced training weeks.

What is so wonderful about Son-Rise is that it is *not even for the child*, who is perhaps content in his protected world of autism. It is for *us*, the parents and families who want a more typical life for our children and who, by realizing this, can decide to turn inward and work on *ourselves*.

Son-Rise is an attitudinal program based on the principles of the Option Process, designed by Barry Neil Kaufman and Samahria Lyte Kaufman even before their autistic child was born. The Option Process comprises a set of practical tools and strategies toward self-help and personal fulfillment. These principles have allowed people worldwide to live happier and more fulfilling lives. It was only through the exploration of these principles of the Option Process that the Kaufmans were able to address their son's autism in such a unique, nonjudgmental way. The Option Process is designed to help us address our attitudes and beliefs in order to become happier people. Therefore, the Son-Rise Program is only effective when we decide to truly confront our own challenges, which in turn allows us to truly be there for our children. Some of the fundamental Option Process principles include the realizations that happiness is a choice, we all have our own answers, our reactions are fueled by our beliefs, and being nonjudgmental is incredibly powerful. We have embarked on this journey together with our volunteers, who have displayed the most incredible open-mindedness and bravery in tackling life-long collections of attitudes and beliefs, initially in the spirit of loving N but ultimately in loving ourselves.

It is so fascinating to me how "talking the talk" doesn't even work. My son can tell when I'm not truly present and letting go of my issues. I have learned that children with autism are so incredibly intuitive and perceptive that it forces us to really confront ourselves if we want to connect with them. I am excited to implement these tools and to attend programs at the Option Institute throughout the rest of my days, even after we move through autism. My husband and I are learning how to be better parents to our younger son as well. Our volunteers, who mostly began as perfect strangers, have joined us to form a most beautiful and connected family. They actually requested weekly group meetings because they are so full of passion and energy for N. Our volunteers noticed that working with N in this process positively impacts their respective weeks. N and our volunteers are my heroes. Watching them each choose happiness over depression, punctuality over tardiness, 3 E's (energy, excitement, and enthusiasm) over boredom, letting go of inhibitions over self-consciousness, love over a judgmental state—the list is endless— has been awe-inspiring for me. It has provided me with limitless hope for N and all of humankind. Their willingness and passion to learn and grow has opened my eyes and restored my faith in the goodness of people and the benevolence of the universe. I feel so incredibly blessed to have the privilege to continue on this most spiritual path with such special individuals.

Best of all is the progress we've seen with N. Since we got back from the Start-Up, we haven't experienced one tantrum. He will now hold our hand and allow us to take him from room to room. He makes more eye contact and is even beginning to show flickers of expression and happiness. Last week, he started pointing to things and verbalizing more. The very same child, who used to have meltdowns when a therapist would arrive, now runs into his volunteers' arms before they can even take off their coats. His volunteers are passionate and love being with him. The change in him is incredible, and we've only just begun! Even if we were never to see another gain from the Son-Rise Program, it would already have been worth every minute and every penny spent toward this effort. This program has given me a relationship with my son again.

I finally feel like we're undoing all the damage we witnessed while he was in school, back when we unknowingly created a scared and untrusting child. I can finally say that the bond we used to have is returning, and our loving son is starting to emerge. I spent a year and a half feeling miserable and sorry for myself having been dealt the "autism card." I've spent hundreds of hours online researching the latest and greatest treatments and interventions wondering which would cure our son. We've dreaded waking up in the morning and yearned for bedtime, day after day, week after week, and month after month for almost two years. And now, at the two year anniversary of our son's autism diagnosis, I am finally happy. I am at peace and excited for the possibilities that lie ahead. I am so fortunate to be connected with the Son-Rise Program and staff. Most of all, I am so fortunate and blessed to have the miracle that is my son.

SAINTED LOVE

When she was four, a parentless child crawled onto my lap and made it clear she wanted to go home with me. Well, maybe not entirely clear as she had no verbal skills. I thought she wanted to go home with her brother, who happened to be sitting next to me and was assigned to a different foster home. When I attempted to clarify what she meant, she shook her head no and pointed right at me. "Ohhhhh, you want to go home with me?" I asked. And that is how our journey began.

Jazmine is the youngest of six children born to a woman who was too devastated by the evils of heroin to know how to be a mother. By the time Jazmine was four, no family members were left to care for the children. The Division of Youth and Family Services (DYFS) had lost patience, and the family faced their final eviction together. I had a tiny bit of insight into this family since the oldest sibling was one of my students. I am a school psychologist in a high school, so when Social Services came to visit him, they had to do it in my presence. He was a proud young man who would rather give his right arm than give away his family secrets, but still, the clues were all there. His wardrobe was limited to one pair of jeans and two T-shirts. As the weather grew colder, he continued to arrive each day without a winter coat. By the time he and his siblings were taken into custody of DYFS, he had learned to trust me, which is why I was the one who accompanied him to his sibling visits at the local DYFS office.

From the first visit, it was clear that his little sister (the only girl of the group) had taken a liking to me. She did not speak but would give one of her rare smiles when she saw me and always greeted me with a running hug. I should not have been surprised when she chose me, but I was. I should not have been surprised when DYFS told me they needed help and asked if I could either take her or two of her brothers for a couple of weeks, but I was. I probably should not have been surprised when they called one night and told me she was going home with me the next day, but again, I was. After all, I wasn't a trained foster parent. Hell, I wasn't even a parent! I was just some woman with a bleeding heart who wanted to help. The time was right. September 11 had just occurred, and what American wasn't willing to help someone in need?

Almost eleven years later, it seems hard to believe but, at the time, I really thought that this was going to be a short-term arrangement. "A few weeks," I was told. "Two months tops." *Okay*, I thought, *I can handle this for a little bit.* In the meantime, I decided to use my knowledge as a child study team case manager to obtain some services for Jazmine. It was obvious that Jazmine had speech delays, so I figured I would start there. Yes, I was that naïve. No matter how capable I thought I was, five years of working in a school and half a lifetime of babysitting and being a nanny could never prepare me for the long road ahead. Little did I know then that by trying to get to the bottom of one weakness I would be opening the door to so many more.

The most shocking part of this time was that not a single person in my life was surprised at my decision to take in this little girl. I am conservative by nature and have fraught over much less life-altering choices. I will never forget the day I went to tell my parents about Jazmine coming to stay with me. I was scared out of my mind for my father's reaction, but his immediate acceptance just cemented my conviction that I was doing the right thing. My mother echoed his feelings and told me that after seeing me with Jazmine at one of her brother's football games, she knew it was inevitable. The truth is, I never really had a choice. The minute she crawled onto my lap, my future was sealed.

A few weeks earlier, I visited this very affected family together with my colleague, a social worker. That was actually the first time I laid eyes on Jazmine. She was just a scared, dirty, hungry little thing who went away when her "mother" told her to. Once we left the visit, my coworker told me she thought my purpose in life was to help families like this and asked if I had ever considered fostering. I had not, but I heard the message my friend was sending. I was single and in my early thirties. She suggested that helping other people's children may have been God's plan for me. I defiantly told her that I thought parenting was a two-person job and that I did not think it was fair to purposefully do that to a child. What child doesn't wish he or she had a mom *and* a dad? Additionally, parenting is hard work and not something easily done by one person. Everyone has bad days, and when you are a single parent, you have no escape. You have no one to hand the child off to when you are at the end of your rope. I made it clear that this was not something I would intentionally do.

How funny that my mind was changed so quickly. Suddenly, I had no concern in my ability to do it alone and a "superwoman/I can save the world" mentality came over me. Not only did I take Jazmine in but I added all five of her brothers to my "to do" list, and my world began to revolve around them.

It was a cold day when DYFS handed Jazmine and a half-filled duffle bag containing stained clothing over to me. I had three of her brothers with me that day, and we were all excited about Jazmine coming to stay with me. She had very few words, but the way she snuggled into me and would not let go spoke volumes. We arrived at my home, and as I showed her around, I immediately noticed that she could not walk up or down stairs. It dawned on me how small she was, and I would later learn the devastating impact of years of neglect and malnutrition. I did not know much about Jazmine and her eating habits. When I asked her brothers what dinner usually consisted of, they told me they ate "quarter cookies" because that was what they could afford. I was not going to serve that for dinner but remembered the home visit just a few weeks earlier when the social worker and I went shopping and brought bags and bags of groceries back to the house. When Jazmine saw the box of waffles, her face lit up. Since this was a sure winner, I planned our first meal to be "breakfast for dinner." I was shocked at how much she ate . . . and the speed at which she did it. I later learned that she was hoarding, which is normal for kids who never knew when their next meal would be. Still naïve, I did not flinch at this, or the fact that between each helping she *needed* a clean plate, or the fact that if I as much as stepped a foot into another room, she was right behind me. Jazmine did not say much, but she watched every move I made and never let me out of her sight.

Becoming a pseudoparent on December 12 makes for a very busy holiday season, and the reality of my decision would not sink in for quite a while. At the time, I was too busy buying little girl clothes and a velvet Christmas dress to really think about what I had done. As soon as the new year began, Jazmine and I started going from evaluation to evaluation to catch up on all of the immunizations and testing she had missed while under the so-called care of Mommy Karen. What I quickly learned was that Jazmine had asthma, triple X syndrome, a submucous cleft palate, an array of developmental delays, and lead poisoning. She had not reached any developmental milestone at an appropriate age. She was a four-year-old in the body of a two-year-old with the speech ability of a child even younger than that. During this same time, we returned to court every two months to hear our fate. Was Jazmine going to be returned to Karen? Would they ask me to keep her? Would they move her to another home? I lived day to day, falling more in love with this child, who called me "Jenn Jenn" and never knowing when our time together would end.

One day, eight months into our journey, Jazmine called me "Mommy." My heart melted. I loved her as I imagined loving a biological child, but she had a mother, and I wanted to respect that. I also did not want to upset her brothers and was uncertain how they would react to Jazmine calling another woman "Mommy." I gently explained that I was just there to help her mommy, and she should continue to call me by the nickname we had established from the beginning. She would do so for a day or two and then sneak in another "Mommy." After a few times, it hit me. All this little munchkin wanted was a mom. For all intents and purposes, I was that person and behaved more like a mom in the eight months we had been together than Karen had in over four years. By not allowing Jazmine to call me Mommy, I was depriving her of a basic need. When I finally stopped correcting her, I did it with fear. I had to be honest and admit that I loved being her mom and hearing that word. But what if I allowed it and then they took her away?

That fear became a distinct possibility at one point while I was fostering Jazmine. I have learned a lot about DYFS over the years, and most of it isn't pretty. I could write a book on this topic alone but will simply say that not all foster parents are what I would describe as suitable. Jazmine's five older brothers lived in countless homes over the years, including shelters, housing projects, a teen center, and the home of a drug dealer. All of the boys were very attached to me and enjoyed spending time with us. Most likely, it had nothing to do with me but was simply due to the fact that I was the only foster parent who planned events for all six kids to be together.

I treated Jazmine and her brothers like children, whereas others treated them like foster children. A few of the foster parents could not understand why I did the things I did or why a single woman would make the choices I did. Much of their lives were based on ulterior motives, so they assumed the same for me. They were certain that I was using Jazmine to get to the teenage boys and that I must have wanted to have sex with them. When the boys told them they were wrong, they still tried everything they could to destroy me. They reported their false claims to DYFS and to the administration of the high school where I work. Meetings were held, investigations were conducted, and I could not breathe. I spent countless hours in the principal's office at my school just sobbing as he would relay yet another lie that was reported to him. I knew I had done nothing wrong, but the accusations alone were enough to kill me. That was when I had my first panic attack. Each time the phone rang, I jumped. What if they took Jazmine away based on a false report alone? Who would take her? Would they be able to manage her medical needs? I could not let that happen.

The investigations proved that I had never done or said anything remotely inappropriate to the boys, and I will forever be grateful to our DYFS caseworker, who may have been the only one to truly believe in me. She promised me that Jazmine was safe in my home, but the fear lingered. Would they let me keep her?

That question remained unanswered for close to a year as I went back to court every two months to hear the judge's orders. Finally, due to Karen's noncompliance in treatment programs and lack of attempts to see or care for her family, the judge moved forward with the termination of parental rights. What a *huge* day for us. This meant that Jazmine's biological parents had absolutely no legal rights over her, and she was free to be adopted. Like all of my earlier decisions, I never really did have a choice, so I moved forward through the adoption process without blinking an eye. All of the questions that should have come to mind did not. Was I really doing this? Was I choosing to be a single parent? What about dating? Could I do this alone? I simply committed with the same naiveté that I had when I offered to help nineteen months prior. This time, though, I was really doing it alone. My parents were in the process of retiring to Florida, and once they left, I would be left alone without another family member in the state. Despite having good friends, your family is your family, and no one has to help you like they do. My parents left for Florida three days before we appeared in court to finalize the adoption. Don't get me wrong; it was still a great day. Jazmine and I were supported in court by her DYFS caseworker and a close friend, but at the end of the day, it was just the two of us. I had just adopted a child without family or a spouse. I was completely on my own. Looking back, I now realize this would become a recurring theme in my life.

It has been almost eight years since I became a mom in the eyes of the law. In those years, I have experienced extreme moments of pride, joy, and the greatest degree of unconditional love possible. In those same years, I have also experienced tragic losses, grief, disappointment, guilt, shame, and embarrassment. Alone. Our journey has required me, under difficult circumstances, to meet with teachers, school administrators, detectives, and attorneys. Alone. People often tell me that I am lucky to be able to make decisions by myself and not have a partner to argue with. I hear the same story time and again of how a husband is just another child to care for. Well, I sure do not feel lucky as I cry myself to sleep or pace the floor at night by myself. I don't feel lucky when I sit alone in a medical office awaiting the results of another round of testing. I don't feel lucky as I visit the prosecutor's office to discuss Jazmine's legal case. Loneliness is both physical and emotional for me with both sides competing to see which will destroy me first. The decision to become a single mom changes all relationships. I no longer fit in with my single friends who lived a carefree existence and whose time was their own as long as they showed up to work on time. I also didn't fit in with the families that surrounded me. I suddenly realized that I lived in a Noah's Ark community where everyone lives two by two. Even my relationship with family members changed. As my focus turned to Jazmine, I was no longer the fun aunt or cousin who could be there for all. It wasn't bad, it was just different, and I was alone.

People are often dismissive to the difficulties of single parenting, especially when you *only* have one child. "How hard can one be?" Well, I can promise that they do not have a child like mine. Jazmine is considered to be "medically fragile." When I was first asked to care for her, I was told she had asthma that required nebulizer treatments, but that is all I was told. After suffering through numerous pneumonia and bronchitis infections, I learned that Jazmine's pulmonary difficulties are far more advanced. Due to prenatal abuse and neglect, her lungs are smaller than expected, and improper medical care in the first few years of her life caused permanent damage to the upper right lobe of her lung. No air moves through this area, and if we cannot keep Jazmine pneumonia free, that section of her lung will have to be removed completely. When she was in first grade, we went through extensive testing for cystic fibrosis (CF). All initial testing— which included x-ray, CAT scan, and sweat tests—proved positive, so we were sent to a geneticist for the all-telling blood work. It took six long weeks to get the results back. I spent many nights during that time just watching her sleep and crying. What would I do if she had it? How could I handle that alone? I cried tears of relief as I was told she was negative for the gene mutation and was simply a carrier. Her diagnosis was bronchiecstasis instead. Although relieved that my baby girl did not have the possibly life-ending CF, brochiecstasis is likewise a serious, life-altering illness. Complications can cause pneumonia, scarring, and a loss of functioning lung tissue. Severe scarring and loss of lung tissue can ultimately strain the right side of the heart, which can lead to a form of heart failure called cor pulmonale. Jazmine is treated with five different medications and vest therapy daily. Since it was important to clear her lungs via the compression vest first thing each morning, suddenly I had to figure out how to start my already early morning even forty-five minutes sooner in order to attend to Jazmine's medical needs. I was already exhausted and unsure of how I was going to do it, but I knew that I would. I had to.

I was fortunate enough during this same time to have made some friends in my community. I was a Girl Scout leader and cheerleading coach for Jazmine, as well as an eager helper on the sidelines at her softball games. Over time, we started socializing quite a bit with the families of her peers and had quite an active social life. Throughout these years, it became obvious that Jazmine was not quite the same as the other kids, and I don't just mean academically. She was socially awkward, and the behavioral difficulties had begun. Looking back, though, I see how lucky we were at the time. Her peers were still too young to make fun of her or call her stupid, or "sped"—a derogatory term for a special education student. Her behaviors had not yet stopped us from getting invited to barbecues and gatherings of friends. It may have been just the two of us, but we were surrounded by some really good people, who at times helped me to forget that we were alone.

Soon after came the time that Jazmine and I would probably both agree was the happiest time for us as a family. I was in my third season coaching her recreation cheerleading team when a girl joined the squad whom Jazmine had played softball with for a few years prior. Her parents were divorced, and after a bit of friendly banter on the sidelines, her dad asked me on a date. I had dated while caring for Jazmine, but I never felt like this before. What we had was mutual and immediate. Although my responsible parent plan was to wait a few months for us to tell the kids, we could not contain our excitement, and they knew within a few weeks. Jazmine fell head over heels for Rob even faster than I did. When he was not with us, she was asking for him. She was happy and wanted him to be the father she never had. For the first time, I felt like I had a true partner.

The weekends Rob cared for his two children, we would all spend together at my house. He would have a big campout with the three kids in the playroom while he gifted me with a peaceful night of sleep in my bed two floors up. He attended back-to-school night and parent conferences with me and was there when Jazmine was diagnosed with seizure disorder and ADHD. Jazmine was never a problem at home, but as her negative behaviors increased at school, he lent a sympathetic ear and strong shoulder to lean on. This was a man who loved me and my daughter for who we were, knew that it was a package deal, and would not have had it any other way. Jazmine begged him to come over after work each night to have dinner and be there to tuck her in. When we would hear him at the door, it would be a race to see who would get to him first, often resulting in a "Jazmine sandwich."

Rob loved being adored by Jazmine, and I finally knew what it felt like to not be alone. I liked it and was content to spend the rest of my life like that. We were making plans for our future. We dreamed of a small beach wedding surrounded by our children and closest friends and family. His daughter and mine would be dressed in flowing white sundresses, while his son would look as cute as a button in his khakis and white shirt. We would all be barefoot as we pledged to join our families forever. We had already met with builders and were busy designing the home of our dreams.

Unfortunately, God had other plans for us.

One Sunday morning, I heard the kids making their way up the steps to my room. I was surprised to hear them. My aunt had died suddenly, so I had just returned from a one-day trip to Miami for the services. Rob begged me to sleep late and promised to keep the kids quiet so I could do so. They opened my door and said, "Daddy's bleeding." I hopped up, assuming I would head downstairs and clean up whatever mess Rob had made. Something must have struck me on my way down because I asked if he was "awake bleeding" or "asleep bleeding." They told me he was asleep, and I arrived to his side to see him lying on his back with some dried up blood going from his nostril towards his ear. My initial thought was that it was not bad, and I would have him fixed up and eating breakfast in no time. When I knelt down to wake him, he felt very cold and clammy, which surprised me. Rob was my portable heater. He was never cold. Again, my mind did not go to the place it belonged, but instead, I assumed he had gotten sick during the night and that caused the clamminess. I began to panic when he did not respond to my touch or voice. My calls got louder, and my voice got shakier as my search for a pulse went unanswered. Surrounded by three children, I begged him to wake up and reached for the phone to dial 911. My next call was to my best friend whose husband advised me to get the kids out of the room and that they were on their way. I called Rob's ex-wife to come over and ushered the three children, all snuggly in their winter PJs, to the living room couch so they could wait for the ambulance to arrive. I returned to Rob's side and pleaded with him to wake up. He didn't. Our lives forever changed that day, and at age 38, Rob was gone.

Jazmine had suffered from abandonment issues since the day I met her. She cried every morning for the first year and a half when I dropped her off at school and refused to take her jacket off when we went anywhere for fear of being left behind. In the blink of an eye, she lost the man she loved most in the world along with her fantasy of being in a real family with two parents who loved her. In some ways, she lost me that day, too. I became a shell of the person I once was and got out of bed only because I had to, not because I wanted to. I went through the motions of daily life but certainly was not living life. Jazmine's issues at school heightened, her fear of abandonment increased, she stopped sleeping, and I had become a fraction of the advocate I had been. People often credit me for saving Jazmine's life, but truthfully, she may have saved mine. She was my purpose for existing after Rob's death, and as hollow as I was, I still was. We continued to be surrounded by a strong network of friends, but that too would shortly unravel. Little did I know then how alone we would feel in only a matter of time.

It first happened with Jazmine and her friends. The pressures of middle school and the social climate there turned Jazmine into a liability. You see, over the years Jazmine has been diagnosed with many conditions that have a direct impact on her social, academic, emotional, and behavioral functioning. In addition to the previously mentioned asthma, bronchiecstasis, lead poisoning, and seizure disorder, Jazmine has fetal alcohol syndrome/effects (FAS/E), ADHD, mitral valve prolapse, and a central auditory processing disorder.

Although it is hard to know what to blame on which diagnoses, Jazmine has a tremendous amount of difficulties. Lead poisoning brings with it behavior or attention problems, reduced IQ, and aggressive behavior. Triple X syndrome is associated with an increased risk of learning disabilities and delayed development of speech and language skills. According to the literature, delayed development of motor skills, weak muscle tone, and behavioral and emotional difficulties are also possible, but these characteristics vary widely among affected females. Unfortunately, Jazmine was one of the incidences that were affected.

FAS/E, although the most difficult to bear, made the most sense to me. The more I read about it, the more I felt like the literature was describing my child. I was angry. The poor innocent children, who did nothing but grow in the womb of an irresponsible, selfish addict, had to face such a difficult life. It was not fair. Among the issues kids with FAS/E face are learning disabilities, trouble getting along with others, impulsivity, aggressiveness, problems talking and listening, longer time to complete tasks, poor judgment, memory problems, poor problem-solving abilities, trouble applying knowledge and higher thinking, problems understanding why something has happened, trouble with time and money management, lack of common sense, ADHD, anxiety, being easily influenced, difficulty predicting and/or understanding consequences, difficulty separating fact from fiction, disobedience, defiance of authority, poor comprehension of social rules and expectations, faulty logic, and low self-esteem. Needless to say, life is hard for these kids, and sadly, Jazmine is just one of many.

Two of the biggest impacts on her daily life are her socially inappropriate behaviors and need for constant supervision. Jazmine does great in a structured setting, but anything unstructured (playground, gym, lunchroom, hallway) causes great difficulty. She did not act like a typical kid, and her "friends" started to shun her. Let's face it, who wants to be connected to the kid who is always doing something wrong? People say they understand, but they don't. They simply look through judgmental eyes and question what the hell you are teaching *that* child and allowing her to do. I have been attacked privately and publicly by other parents time and again for Jazmine's behaviors. It broke my heart as I saw her four- or five-year-long relationships dissolve before my eyes. I continued to host parties in hopes of assisting her with making and keeping friends. Once a month, I would choose a theme and plan a party around that. For example, in October, we would paint pumpkins, and in December, we would bake cookies. Those parties started becoming the only time Jazmine saw her peers during the month, and then, even those invitations started to be declined. The only time she saw the friends with whom we used to do just about everything was when it was at an event that included entire families. Jazmine never spent time on her own with the girls she had once been inseparable from. However, over time, the invitations to family events stopped, too.

Most of the people on whom I leaned the most as I struggled with Rob's death were no longer in our world. At first, I wanted to understand what had happened and why we were no longer included. Then I realized it did not matter, and I had to accept it. It was another loss, and we were alone again. I did not have time to mourn those losses. I did not have time to fall apart again. Jazmine needed me, and I needed to stay focused for my girl.

I can't say that we did not have anyone in our lives, because we did. I have friends who have stood by me through thick and thin and accept Jazmine for exactly who she is. The very same friends who were my first call after 911 are still very much a part of our lives. We have developed new friendships over time, but it was devastating to watch certain groups of people continue their friend-ships and fun without us. To be dismissed by those who had been my rock was painful and lonely beyond words. It hit me what a solitary life I had chosen when I adopted Jazmine. Although she has the kindest heart I have ever met and is the absolute love of my life, she engages in behaviors that others do not have to tolerate, so they walk away. I do not understand why she does the things she does, and I doubt I ever will.

Being her mom has made me feel like the biggest failure. It pains me that I cannot "fix" her no matter how hard I try. And try I have.

I took her to every specialist and therapist that I could find. I listened to every word the doctors said, followed their advice, and gave her all the medications they suggested. We had charts at home; she had charts at school. I followed every behavior modifica-tion technique I was given, but regardless of the rule or impend-ing consequence, something always went wrong. I felt as if I could not protect Jazmine from herself, and suddenly my goals for her changed. I went from being focused on increasing her academic skills to concentrating on three simple things: keep her out of jail, keep her off the streets, and keep her from getting pregnant. One of her specialists suggested to us what I thought would be the holy grail of help. I was thrilled. This was not a program open to the public, but I was assured that it would be of great help to us. The criteria for placement was strict, and the kids had to have significant needs to be accepted. I met with the program coordinator for the hour-long intake to discuss Jazmine's background, needs, etc. At the end, this woman just looked at me with tears in her eyes and said she could not help me. What? This was the place that helped the kids who could not be helped anywhere else. How could this be? Was my child that far gone? No answers. Just a dead end. I believe that she felt bad but did not want to waste my time and hope when she did not think the program could be effective. As I was leaving, she looked at me with a tear rolling down her face and asked if she could hug me.

During this same time, I was experiencing medical issues myself that needed to be addressed. Like Jazmine, I spent my life visiting doctors and was all too familiar with waiting rooms due to the diagnosis of Addison's disease as a child. Although life was not complication free, it was managed on daily mediations and by taking precautions. Suddenly though, I was facing new and unfamiliar fears. I was advised to live a healthier and less stressful life. I was a single mom of a daughter suffering from multiple disabilities, and I worked full time. My life was not about taking care of me. It was first and foremost about taking care of Jazmine. After her came my job, my home, and the teams I coached. It was not as if I had people lining up to assist me or the monetary resources to hire help. How was this going to be possible?

I was tired, hopeless, and alone. I was not good at asking for help. The last time I truly allowed someone to be a part of our lives and share my responsibilities, he left us. People had good intentions of helping, but at the end of the day, they all had their own families to worry about. Very few people actually meant it when they said, "Call anytime." I learned that relying on others equaled disappointment. I had many sleepless nights, so I would amuse myself with Facebook. Like many, Facebook has given me the opportunity to reconnect with many people from my past. About two years ago, I got into a conversation with some women I had gone to college with. I was always so impressed with one in particular and her ability to be an open book about what she goes through with her son's autism. I have never been good at putting things "out there" and certainly would not publicize Jazmine's issues on Facebook. Not that I think my friend was wrong, but Jazmine is older and has peers on Facebook. I would not want to cause her further humiliation by having her peers read my updates on her progress.

That one conversation with my college friend, who you have come to know as Goddess, changed my life though. Little did I know that I was speaking to one of the greatest Thinking Moms I would have the pleasure of knowing. Goddess told me that she had an appointment with a homeopath who had a reputation of doing wonderful things with children who were diagnosed with all sorts of disorders. He had a waiting list, so she suggested I make an appointment, knowing I could always cancel. I did so and marveled over the next few months as my friend continued to share story after wonderful story about her son's progress.

Over those same months, Jazmine and I faced situation after horrible situation, which just cemented to me how severely in need she was of serious intervention. More medication was suggested, and I had to put my foot down and say no. A stimulant for the ADHD was acceptable. An SSRI for depression and anxiety, I dealt with. It was better than the bloody fingers she used to have from the constant picking. However, I was not going to allow her to take an antipsychotic medication. I did not believe she needed it, nor did her neurologist. I knew my appointment with the homeopath was approaching, so I just held my breath and hoped for the best.

When I finally met the homeopath, I had no idea what to expect, and I do not think I am even able to describe that experience all these months later. As I mentioned earlier, I am conservative by nature, so homeopathy was pretty out there for me. My goal was to leave no stone unturned in my quest to help my daughter. I left his office thinking that I had either just handed a ton of money I could not afford over to a quack who took advantage of desperate parents, *or* I had just met my very own personal Wizard of Oz. Even though I have days when it could go either way, what I can tell you is that our lives have improved dramatically since that day.

Yes, we have seen some solid improvements since starting to take a homeopathic remedy, but that is not the best part. The best part is the community of people that have since embraced us. After our initial consultation, Goddess offered me membership to a private group on Facebook, whose members are other parents who are all struggling to recover their children. The majority are facing autism as their enemy, but they accepted me and recognized that although our labels are different, we shared so many of the same struggles. I will never forget the day I officially entered the group. Goddess posted a message on the group's wall, asking everyone to welcome me. Just seeing that message and the posts that followed opened the floodgates to tears I did not even know I had. They came hard, and they came fast. At times, I could not breathe, because the sobs were uncontrollable. Until I was welcomed to this group, I did not realize how alone I had truly been in all of this. Or at least, I could not admit it. I had stopped talking about Jazmine and her issues because I did not want to scare anyone else off. I was often told how strong I was. It was a farce. I was not strong. I was hiding behind a wall of shame and secrets, too afraid to connect with my feelings for fear of falling apart again and never coming out of it. I had been keeping it all to myself but did not have to anymore. I was not alone. I was *not* alone. I *was not alone.* Wow. It was an extremely powerful moment in my life.

This group, this wonderful place in cyberspace reminds me of the TV show *Cheers*. A familiar, comfortable place where you can just be yourself and where everyone knows your name. The only difference is that our special place is just ours. We all have nicknames. I had the honor of being named Saint. Although I am certainly far from the real deal, it touches my heart that this group of virtual strangers could recognize my intentions as being good and pure. To be honest, the real Saint is my girl—but for now, I'll keep the name warm for her.

Since the first day I was welcomed into this group, I have shared the good, the bad, and the ugly with them. I do not think I have ever faced such unconditional love and support in my life. The group members are warm and creative and smart. We talk about our kids, but we also just talk—and laugh. I am not embarrassed by what Jazmine does, and I do not have to worry about disappointing them when I share yet another horror story with them. All of these parents struggle yet cheer for one another. We celebrate each stride another's child makes, while mourning together the setbacks another faces. We may sympathize when we read a post, but we are never shocked. Behaviors that I would once have been too ashamed to speak of, I can easily tell our group. Nobody judges, and they understand in a way that parents of neurotypical kids are unable to.

I am a healthier individual for having them in my life and a better parent for knowing them. To be honest, I am in awe of them. Homeopathy brought them to me, but they have led me towards so many other possibilities. I am slowly learning about all of the treatments—including HBOT, chelation, homotoxicology, and sublingual immunotherapy—available to me, and I will not stop until I find the right one or combination for my girl. I have been posing questions to the medical community for almost ten years. Little did I know that only when I stopped listening would I hear so much.

I started this chapter by telling how our journey began. Although I would like to know how it turns out, this is not the end. Our journey is far from over, and I will be encountering behavioral, academic, and medical problems with Jazmine throughout our lives. The difference is now I am not alone, and with the Thinking Moms by my side, I never will be again.

Bytes from the Count

Just tell me! Show me! What do I have to do? Even if I can't implement it, at the very least I want to know what the solution is. At least then I would have a definitive plan. Do I have to move this ten-story building by hand? Is that the answer? Great! At least I know what to do now! It will take me a lifetime to do it myself, so let me get started right away. At least I know the answer now and there's an end and a way to get there.

By the way, only an idiot would move things by hand. Let me design some tools to make it easier and faster.

GODDESS DEFIES GRAVITY

Something has changed within me; something is not the same
I'm through with playing by the rules of someone else's game
Too late for second guessing; too late to go back to sleep
It's time to trust my instincts, close my eyes and leap . . .
It's time to try defying gravity . . .
—WICKED (THE MUSICAL)

I was sitting at the kitchen table in my college apartment with my roommates discussing some drunken escapades from the night before when the discussion turned to two friends who were dating. We wondered whether they would make it long term. Ever the optimist, I voted yes. My bestie and roommate sized up the length of the table and placed a saltshaker in the middle. "Okay, this saltshaker is normal people—reality." Because, you know, in college a saltshaker can be just about anything. Then she took an ashtray and put it midway on the optimist side of the saltshaker and said, "This is me." She then took the peppershaker and put it just to the left side of the line and compared it to one of our slightly pessimistic roommates.

"And you," she continued while picking up a coffee mug, "are here," and her voice trailed off as she took the mug, pushed it to the far edge of the optimist side of the table, reconsidered, walked through the kitchen, through the living room, and to the very edge of the apartment, and placed the mug on the floor. We all laughed about it, but for the past few years, I have thanked God every day that I live in my own somewhat delusional, positively feelin', groovy, optimisticky kind of place. I've needed every ounce of that optimism because there have been days when that's been the only thing left to cling to.

Funny thing about college then and life now. I feel like I am relearning so many things that I intuitively knew back then. I knew myself a lot better. My mind wasn't cluttered with balancing a real job and responsibilities, or with buying things I *had* to have . . . like insanely expensive purses, sunglasses, and shoes. I knew what was really important to me then, and I was true to myself and my beliefs. I had a bug jar and caught stray spiders and put them outside. I read new age-y books and became a vegetarian (didn't last though). I was generally kind to people. I mean, sure, we had parties and charged at the door to cover spring wardrobes, but that was nothing like the consumerism I came to embrace while living in New York City and working next door to Bergdorf's. I feel like in the years that followed college, as I made more money and became more sophisticated, I forgot my own core values and what was really important to me. Though I will not argue that rooms full of furniture from Bloomingdale's don't trump my sponge-painted This End Up furnished apartment; in some ways I had more back then than I did in my early thirties.

This leads me to the state of mind I was in when I had my children. We had the cutest nursery for G, my oldest. When the twins came along, my daughter R and my son Harry, they also got an amazing nursery decorated to absolute perfection. My kids paraded around in Ralph Lauren footies, Kingsley, and Baby Dior. I spent months deliberating diaper bags: the LV or the funkier Suzy by Hammitt USA? I was obsessed. It was just all so cute. When we met our pediatrician, who looked like she just stepped out of a dressing room at Barney's, I was sold. I did everything she said without question. It's only now that I can look back and see what a fucking idiot I was. Avoiding tuna but taking a mercury-laden flu shot while pregnant? Sign me up! Rhogam while pregnant? Sure! Why not? Hep B shot in the hospital the day Harry was born, which was four weeks early, weighing in at a whopping 4.4 lb.? Bring it on! Oh, he got jaundice? Obviously unrelated. Head swelling and scream-ing after the DTaP? Heads sometimes just grow faster, right? Big head, big brain! Reflux, projectile vomiting, 24/7 crying? Relax, all babies go through that. *What the fuck was I thinking?* Oh yeah, I was thinking how cute the pediatrician would think the twins were in their matching Jacadi outfits. Asshole I was.

Harry was born tiny but healthy and went home with me after our forty-eight-hour stay. He and R were perfect. They both tracked objects, gazed at us, held their heads up, cooed at us, smiled at us . . . just perfect. And then, things started going wrong. When I look at the pediatric records now, all the puzzle pieces are there. Why couldn't I see what was happening at the time?

After Harry's four-month visit, his head got bigger and big-ger—sixtieth percentile head size in a child who was in the less than third percentile for height and weight. He cried all day long and projectile-vomited every ounce of formula (of course formula) that we gave him. After his six-month visit, Harry was gone. He still did the physical things. He crawled and walked, but he stopped responding to us. And yet, I kept going with vaccines for another entire *year* before I stopped. If I had only paused to think a bit, the "college me" would have put the whole thing together. The "thirty-four-year-old me" crammed fur-covered earmuffs over her ears. Realistically, after countless rounds of antibiotics, ear tubes, and hearing screenings, I was sitting at an eleven-month-old's early intervention evaluation already knowing something was really wrong. I was treating autism by the time he was thirteen months old, just without an official diagnosis. The diagnosis came later, at around nineteen months. By then I knew what the diagnosis would be, and I walked into that developmental pediatrician's office know-ing what he would say. Knowing didn't make it any easier.

For the record, here is what Asshat (the pediatrician) said, "Autism. Not much you can do. Behavioral programs to manage him as he grows older. He may talk; he may not. More than likely, an apraxia diagnosis down the road. Join a support group to get through it." I didn't really process what he was saying. I am not sure I have fully processed it two years later.

Process it or not, I am one of those people who "do" things. I don't sit around and wait for things to change. I make the change I want. I'm also a reader, and months before the appointment, I had started trying to figure it all out. I had a daughter who hit every milestone early. She babbled "mamadadababa" before she was seven months old. I now had a son who cried and threw up all day long. I started asking Asshat questions about all the things I'd read over the last few months. "What about special diets . . . ?" "Oh, they don't help. Waste of time." "What about that thing people do to remove mercury . . . chelation (only I pronounced the *ch* like you would in Chelsea) . . . ?" "Not safe, kids die." He patted me on the back for starting speech and occupational therapy so early and sent me on my way. I left and vowed never to give Asshat another penny.

I had a good-size friends list on Facebook. That night, I simply typed "autism" into my status. It was all I could manage. I have the most amazing family and friends on the planet. I really, really do. The outpouring of love and support that night is something that I will never, ever forget. I looked back at the comments from that status many more times than I could count. My family and friends carried me through that first dark year, and I do mean carried. But something changed in me that night. I resolved that I would do what it took, whatever it took, to recover Harry from autism. After all, I was beginning to see that I did this to him. I would spend the rest of my life undoing it if I had to.

So, I bought books, and I read books. Book after book after book. Books by biomedical doctors, books on all kinds of treatments for autism, books by parents of kids with autism. I read books every spare second I had, and when I wasn't reading books, I was online, Googling, joining Yahoo! groups, scouring the Talk About Curing Autism (TACA) website for anything and everything I could possibly do for Harry. We went gluten-free, casein-free (GFCF) cold turkey. The day after we removed milk, Harry turned to his name for the first time since he was a baby. He looked at us briefly. The lights were on. He fell down, scraped his knee, and cried. That was significant because he never cried when he got hurt. It was like he was starting to feel pain. Harry's reflux disappeared forty-eight hours after we went GFCF, so we removed the megadose of Prevacid he was taking. Progress.

The diet worked. That compelled me to seek out other treatments that would work, too. We brought a special-needs nutritionist on board because the only things Harry ate prior to going GFCF were milk, yogurt, cheerios, and gyro meat. We went organic and stopped using harsh chemicals and pesticides. We started oral-motor therapy for apraxia. We started physical therapy, got in to see a DAN! (Defeat Autism Now!) doctor and started the DAN! protocol. After we'd started these treatments, I took Harry back to our glam doc for a sick visit. I refused his flu shot and got pissed when the doctor rolled her eyes at me when I described what happened on "the diet." Then I fired the dipshit and her Louboutins. It kills me now how many times I brought up the fact that Harry didn't react well to milk only to have her dismiss it. I could have prevented so much pain if I had listened to my gut. Guess what? The pediatrician doesn't have to live with your child or the consequences: You do. Trust your instincts. They're all you've got.

I realized I was through listening to doctors who got their continuing education from an endless stream of pharmaceutical reps who marched into their offices. (Ours was also a spokesperson for Similac . . . I mean, really.) We found a different pediatrician off the askdrsears.com site, who dressed in mom jeans, was open-minded, and ran all the blood work we asked of her. We were on our way. We also got in to see one of the best biomedical doctors in the country. We tested Harry's urine and stool and discovered that he had bacteria in his gut called clostridia, which was common for kids with autism. The presence of clostridia was the source of his huge distended belly and unending constipation. We treated it first with antibiotics and antifungals, and then later really healed it with homeopathy. We discovered Harry had a thyroid problem and treated that, too. We started antioxidant supplements to help lower oxidative stress, which he had tested very high for. We also gave methyl–B12 injections combined with DMG, folinic acid, fish oil, and vitamin E (which we thought might help him to speak). We started hyperbaric oxygen therapy and a list of countless other behavioral interventions to try to bring Harry back to us. I was at war with myself, asshole doctors, pharmaceutical companies, and autism. And I was going to win.

Somewhere in there, in the dark year when Harry was between age one and a half and two and a half, I realized that I would never be able to go back to the way I was before . . . and I didn't really want to. It felt good to spend my money on important things. (That feeling is gone by the way, right along with my healthy bank account. It has been replaced by credit cards complete with balances.) I remembered who I was. I remembered where I came from. I will never forgive myself that Harry had to be my reminder, but that voice I ignored that questioned *vaccine-preservatives-while-pregnant* right before the nurse jabbed me with the flu shot sings strong in my head now, and I listen.

At a certain point, I found I had to put all the anger and regret aside. It's still there simmering and will have its use one day, but most days I find that for me, it takes more energy to hold on to it. I need that energy to recover my child and to *believe* that I will do so even when he runs endlessly back and forth, stimming with his hands and screaming, "Ahhhh," for what seems like unending periods of time.

But I digress.

By age two and a half, we were a year into the biomed leap with Harry. We started to do other things and tried other methods, shifting focus away from prescription drugs and toward classical homeopathy. We saw some big gains, such as both sides of Harry's body working together. One of the biggest gains at the time was that he could finally jump. Encouraged by the progress, I started looking into the CEASE protocol pioneered by Tinus Smits. We found a CEASE homeopath and started clearing toxins. Our first clear was the flu vaccine that I got while pregnant. The clear brought on detox rashes that covered Harry's body on and off for ten weeks, but he made more gains. His auditory processing delay decreased significantly. Next, we started viral testing and discovered that his nagalese level was elevated. This meant that Harry's body was not able to recognize or fight viruses that caused immune system issues much like those that a cancer or AIDS patient suffers. We found another amazing autism doctor, started GcMAF, got more detox rashes, and saw huge gains. Once we began treating the viral issues, Harry's cognition was at warp speed. His receptive language began to explode. At four, he could spell his name. He knew how to read sight words. He began nodding yes and no. It was all so exciting.

As this was going on, my dad took over cooking for Harry, researching every nutrient he needed and what food to add to get it in him. My dad, or Papou as he is called, has an amazing bond with my son. They play games on the computer, practice signing, and eat together. Harry loves him deeply, and we are so fortunate to have him and my mom as a daily part of Harry's life. Equally helpful, my mom took over oral-motor therapy and did the exercises with Harry twice a day. She also shuttled him to therapy appointments, taught him how to pedal a tricycle, and took him swimming, building his confidence and strength.

My husband's parents lived further away at that point but offered their love, understanding, and crucial (and I do mean crucial) financial support so we could put Harry in an integrated classroom with an one-to-one aide. They also helped pay for treatments we wanted to try. They asked questions and became involved. They made a real effort to connect with Harry, never treating him differently than his brother and sister, and because of that he is close with them as well. He loves tickles from Nana and roughing up from Papa. His aunts and uncles are amazing, too. We are so lucky to have supportive family members. They have never once undermined anything we've tried to do. For any grandparents out there reading this, please realize that it truly takes a village. Offer whatever support you can. Babysit. Buy the affected child in your life an iPad. Get involved with treatments. Your children will never forget how you pulled through for them in their time of need. Don't judge, just listen. And help, help, help.

Somewhere in there, we started VBA/ABA, which gave Harry a way to communicate with us. We moved so he could attend one of the premier schools in the country, which was full of caring, gentle teachers and therapists who loved him. Truly loved him.

I began mentoring the parents of newly diagnosed children to help them see that there was a light of hope in this dark tunnel. Our kids can and do get better. I started a Facebook page called "Healing Harry," on which I chronicled all of Harry's gains and developments, so that my wonderful friends and family could easily see his progress, ask questions, and become informed.

Through all of this, my husband worked, and worked, and worked, and is still working to try to support all of our efforts to heal our child. We leapt together, both believing that Harry was just trapped behind the complex symptoms we collectively call autism, and we work as a unit to try to resolve those symptoms one by one, using the other as a sounding board when determining what to tackle next, what will bring speech, what will bring vitality.

Harry is four now, and he is miles from where we started. He is a sweet little boy who loves toys, his siblings, and learning. He is no longer in pain and is no longer constipated. He can sit in restaurants, behaves properly in stores, and is great on an airplane. He loves running and jumping, two things he could not do before homeopathy. He is like a beam of light in our world. He has a smile that captivates me. We still have a long way to go. Harry is still preverbal, although he is signing consistently now and attempting garbled sentences. He is trying to sing. He is getting great at answering questions by pointing and nodding, has great eye contact, and follows directions really well. The light at the end of the tunnel is there.

His twin sister and older brother love him fiercely. They have started asking questions about why he doesn't talk yet. I am not sure what to tell them. Do I tell them he has autism? How much longer will he have it? What is it anyway? How do I begin to explain that he got very sick and his brain got hurt but that every day he is getting better and better? How do I explain that what they will hear as they grow up is not true? Autism is really a medical condition. If it wasn't, there wouldn't be so many recovered kids walking around. In my opinion, there isn't some elusive cause; it all comes down to toxins and how many a particular individual can handle at a particular point in time.

Every day Harry is more "with it" and more "in it" than he was the day before. We will beat this. I know it to the very core of my being. So we keep going forwards, sometimes sideways, sometimes after a step back, but ultimately in the right direction to give him health and happiness.

Remember Asshat, the developmental pediatrician? Thank goodness I didn't listen to most of his advice, but it turns out that he did have one good thought after all. I could never picture myself at a support group meeting. At the time, I was judgmental. What was it? A group of people sitting around crying over autism? Obviously, not for me. But I was wrong. Support groups come in all forms. I think good support is a key factor in recovery from autism because autism is a hard battle to fight. Even with the best practitioners in the country fighting right alongside you, it is a really hard, mostly uphill kind of fight. You need people with you in the trenches who can help you cover enemy fire (e.g., "What do I say to the lady in the store who just gave me a dirty look and told me to control my child?"). You need people who will show you how to dig your foxhole (e.g., "How do I make sure my child has the best possible IEP, and how do I make sure it is adhered to?"). You need people who can help you reload your rifle (e.g., "What are you doing now? What is working for you?"). And you need people who understand your war strategy, who will raise a victory flag along with you when you reach a milestone. It's crucial.

I never did make it to a local meeting, but through what I believe had to be divine intervention, I managed to find the most supportive moms (and dad) on the planet, and we formed a group so tight that we are family. We visit each other as we travel the country to doctor appointments, which we sometimes plan to occur on the same day so we can spend time together with our families. Destination appointments . . . How trendy. We support each other through setbacks, send supplements when needed. We know each other's children, what they're up to, what they like, and when their birthdays are. We hang out at AutismOne and National Autism Association conferences. We sit together cramming presentation information by day, and we sing wine-fueled karaoke at night. We come from all walks of life, all religions, different states, and different countries. But we are like-minded in that we believe in recovery and that our kiddos will get there. Positive thinkers. We lift each other up and support each other. We share our notes, our research, our treatments, our testing. Ultimate optimists, our coffee mugs *all* sitting on the outer edge of my old college apartment. Some of our kids have already recovered or are quite close to it. Some are still fighting their way out. But they will all get there, and so will we. Alone, any one of us could fly, but together, we defy gravity.

SUNSHINE'S SONG

Oh, if this little light of mine
Combined with yours today,
How many watts could we luminate?
How many villages could we save?
—JASON MRAZ

"How can this be happening? Yesterday this kid was perfect and had sunshine shooting out of his ass. Today he has autism!"

"Aw, honey," my mom said to me in her most calm and loving voice, "Sunshine will shoot out of his ass again. I am sure of it."

★　★　★

Rob has been and always will be the "golden child" of the family. As the first grandchild for both sets of grandparents, the day when he arrived was probably the happiest of all our lives. We had planned on waiting until fall before trying to get pregnant, but like so many of our plans in life, things have a way of changing. Something had changed instantly for me. Even though it was only the beginning of August, I just *knew* it was time to start trying. I am not sure I can even explain the feeling I had, but I was certain that it was time.

Jon had just started working in Philadelphia, and the day after I got knocked up I took a walk all over the city. It was a beautiful, sunny day, and I walked for miles. I ate a greasy cheese steak, poked around in shops, went to Ben Franklin's grave, and got some pizza at Lorenzo's. I made all the important stops I had been missing from my years growing up across the river in New Jersey. Wait a minute. Ben Franklin's grave? Sounds odd, I know. Having grown up outside of Philly, I knew the legend of Ben Franklin's final resting place. Rumor has it that if you make a wish and throw a penny on Ben Franklin's grave, your wish will come true. Well, I wished for Rob. I didn't know it would be Rob at the time, but I wished for a baby. I wished to be pregnant. I wished for him. True to form, Ben Franklin delivered. Nine months later, I delivered the most beautiful birthday present my husband Jon will ever receive: his son.

Jon and I met when we were eighteen years old. He was one of the first people I met at college because he was in the same program of studies as my freshman roommate. We became fast friends, and I adored him instantly. We had the same core group of friends throughout our four years at school, but that is all we were for years: just friends. I don't even know when the switch was flipped, but suddenly, during the start of senior year, all I could think about was Jon. We were both single, something that had never happened in the previous three years, and we were always together. Since Jon was a gentleman, I decided to take matters into my own hands. I got drunk and kissed him. I knew instantly that it was the last first kiss I would ever have. I haven't looked back since, and I haven't doubted for a minute that I landed the best guy on the planet.

When we graduated, we moved in together. A year later we got engaged and had the best wedding imaginable. I hate to brag, but our wedding really was perfect. It was not because everything went according to plan either. There were glitches and problems and all the craziness that goes along with every wedding. We just didn't care. We were in love, and all we wanted was a wonderful party with great friends. And that is what we got. I have cried at weddings ever since.

We moved to Chicago just months before we got married, and proceeded to have the best years of our lives. Jon was working hard at his career, and I went back to school and got my master's degree in education. We met amazing friends and had a blast. We lived it up for three fabulous years in the Windy City, and we both still feel like that town is our home.

Jon got transferred back to the East Coast, and we settled into a more grown-up life. I was teaching, and we were saving all we could for a down payment on a house. We decided to plan a two-week vacation and camped along the Washington, Oregon, and California coastline and got to experience the type of getaway that is impossible once children come along. It was our last vacation before I became pregnant. It was the end of our carefree days, and I will never forget it.

Jon and I had planned our life perfectly. We got pregnant with no problems at all. This was such a blessing as I watched so many friends struggle with fertility problems. Other than the fact that I was totally wiped out and tired every second of the day for the first three and a half months, there was absolutely nothing remarkable about our pregnancy. This was the most loved and wanted child on the planet, and we couldn't wait for him to arrive. We didn't know if we were having a boy or a girl, but this baby was due two days before Jon's birthday, and my husband was 100 percent convinced that he or she was going to be born on that very day. I thought he was nuts. What were the odds of that actually happening?

We bought a new house in New Jersey and settled in five days before Rob was born. The day after our due date, I went to Philadelphia with Jon, dropped him off at work, and went to get my driver's license. The thought of hanging out at the DMV with a brand new baby made me want to stick knitting needles in my eyes, so I decided to get it done before the baby came. Please, don't get your driver's license photograph taken when you are nine months pregnant. I mean it; don't do it. In my photograph, I looked like

I had eaten an entire McDonald's franchise. I felt awful and tired that day, so I went to our new home while Jon was finishing up work and took a nap on the empty floor. I picked him up, and off we went to the OB appointment. The doctor said she would see us in a week if nothing happened, but Jon had other plans. He told me the baby was coming the next day on his birthday and that we were going out for some spicy Mexican food to help matters along. Come on! That doesn't actually work! But I humored him anyway. Our waiter brought the spiciest salsa they had. We got home, and I didn't feel well, so I went to bed at nine. I was up at midnight and couldn't go back to sleep. I felt just awful. The next day at 1:16 p.m. on Jon's birthday, our baby boy was born. He was healthy and alert and just as beautiful as he could possibly be. We were a family.

Things were perfect! We had a new home in a neighborhood we loved, and we had the most beautiful baby on the planet. People stopped me in stores to tell me how beautiful he was. The kid was—and still is—unbelievably gorgeous. Oh, and he was smart! He was able to tell me all the letters that were on the refrigerator at fifteen months. Sweet, cute, and smart? What a bonus! Of course we had to do this again, and right on cue, I got the same feeling that we absolutely had to get pregnant again immediately. Two weeks later, the stick turned pink, and we were going to have another baby. Life could not be any better. The trouble was that in all that perfect happiness something was happening to the golden child, and we were living with our heads in the sand.

Sometime around nine months old, Rob started getting ear infections. He had his first one at Christmas time. He was tired and had a fever. We brought him to the pediatrician. According to his doctor, he needed a broad-spectrum antibiotic. Of course, we listened to our wise doctor, and Rob's ear infection went away. You can probably guess that this would not be our last tangle with ear infections. Rob had a boatload of them. Each and every ear infection was treated diligently with antibiotics. I don't even know how many rounds of antibiotics he received from nine months to age four, and I am not sure I want to go back through his records to find out. The antibiotics completely wrecked his digestive system because they kill all of the good bacteria in the gut as they are fighting the unwanted bacteria that cause the infection. Sadly, at the time I had no idea that this was happening. I mean, I was the best mommy on the planet! We promptly went to the doctor for each and every illness, we finished all of our antibiotics, and we vaccinated right on schedule. I know that he got vaccines while he was sick, and I know that he got them while he was on antibiotics. Rob's digestive health began to deteriorate quickly. He stopped gaining weight, and he stopped growing at the rate he should have been. He developed horrible diarrhea that would burn his backside to the point of bleeding. It looked like his tiny bottom was dipped in boiling water. He had very small appetite. However, he was insanely sweet and happy, and because he was meeting all his milestones, our pediatrician wasn't concerned. Things started to change. The changes were subtle and slow, and no one really noticed them, but we were taken off the happy family superhighway and put on the autism trail with no map or compass. We were living the dream and had no clue that we had even left the comfort of the paved road.

For some, autism comes into their lives like a bull in a china shop, instantly tearing up the place. One minute a family has a healthy, happy baby, and the next—no words, no smiles, no eye contact. Autism entered our world like a cat burglar. It was quiet and sneaky, and slowly started stealing things from us without us noticing. Hmmm, Rob is quiet today. Wow, no weight gain again at this visit? Gee, Rob loves to carry that one book around all day. Did you hear that? He can recite *The Lorax* . . . the whole book! That was our first red flag. At two and a half years of age, he had the entire book memorized (remember, he's smart . . . the whole book at two) and would walk around repeating pages out of the book. We thought it was odd behavior, so we went to the pediatrician. She really didn't think we had any reason for concern and told us that "in her heart of hearts" she felt he would be just fine. She also said that we should take him to a developmental pediatrician "just to be sure." Whew, what a relief! He is just very bright, maybe even gifted. We will take him to a specialist, and she'll confirm what we already know.

After a few months on a waiting list, we went to the developmental pediatrician. It was our first trip out of the house in underwear because over the last few months Rob had learned to use the potty! We really felt like winners having him potty trained by three. The doctor observed him, got information from us, and told us that she agreed with the pediatrician. She didn't feel comfortable giving Rob any of the autism labels and felt that he was going to be just fine. She rattled off the names of all the great and wonderful people who had autism, such as Bill Gates, Dan Aykroyd, and of course, Albert Einstein. She acted like we had hit the lottery. We had hit the lottery with him! He was the golden boy and pretty perfect in every way possible. Then she suggested that we contact Early Intervention to get him evaluated—again, "just to be sure."

So we moved onward with more evaluations. This seemed like a lot of evaluations for a kid who was just fine! The Early Intervention team came right before nap (brilliant timing), and Rob was not on his game. Over the course of the testing, they saw that Rob was meeting his age-appropriate benchmarks. He happened to refuse to pick up a crayon and draw, so they fudged the numbers a bit and got him in the program based on a fine-motor delay. Because he was almost three, we were only going to receive a month of services before we would be turned over to the school system. At our meeting with the evaluation team at school, they all seemed very confused as to why we were there. They all watched Rob play with a puzzle and sit like a perfect angel. Most of them felt there was no need to do any further testing. Finally, the speech therapist spoke up and suggested that Rob be tested—"just to be sure." One of the phrases I have grown to despise is "just to be sure." The news was not great. His verbal abilities were below what they should be by over a year. He was going into the special education system.

At my insistence, he started out in a regular preschool with support from the public school special education teachers. It was a great program, in which the public school teamed up with a private preschool and provided a teacher and aides assigned to that particular program. These teachers worked with Rob and other students with delays in a typical setting. There was one problem with this wonderful school. Rob was not thriving in this environment. The teachers could not get him to engage with them or the other students. Rob spent the majority of the time off on his own. "He has autism," they told us. "He needs a more structured program." This was like a punch in the gut. He went to the public school and was placed in a self-contained preschool program after the Christmas break. I sobbed at the meeting. I was angry on the phone when I talked to my mom. I cried to Jon. We talked a lot and came to the only reasonable conclusion: Rob would be just fine. Of course he would! Denial is not just a river in Egypt, you know.

Did I mention we were moving? Jon had to start his new job in Washington, D.C. at the same time we were having the "A" bomb dropped on our hearts. He moved to D.C. in December, while we stayed behind and waited and waited and waited to sell our house. During this time, Rob's brother potty-trained before he was two years old and made leaps and bounds developmentally. Everything about this kid was advanced. And Rob? It was like he was frozen in time, stuck in a block of ice. Some kids regress into autism. Rob seemed to just stop developing, trapped in some kind of autism quicksand. But he was going to be just fine, and I had to focus on selling the house and getting us all to Virginia so we could be together. Six months later, when Rob was four and his brother was two, we moved from New Jersey to Virginia.

New house, new neighborhood, new school, and Rob was still stuck in his time warp. We were seeing little to no progress. When we were still in New Jersey, I had a few people tell me to look into vitamin B12 shots, or to see a doctor who specializes in biomedical interventions for autism. Really? What for? Look at him! He was perfect. Besides, my doctors all told me vaccines don't cause autism. He was just quirky because he was so smart. Yet there he was, halfway through the year and, again, there was no progress to be had.

Slowly, I started to wake the hell up. It was time to start doing something different to help this kid. I found the TACA-USA Yahoo! group and started reading. I searched the Autism Research Institute (ARI) website and found a biomedical doctor who was close by. I will preface what comes next by saying that not all doctors who specialize in biomedical interventions are created equal. Get opinions and do your homework. I promise you it is worth the effort you put into it.

I had decided to take the plunge and go see what all this biomedical stuff was about. This turned out to be both a huge mistake and a huge blessing all rolled into a creepy few months of seeing this doctor. The suggestions given to us were all overboard, and the things she was telling us to do didn't make sense to me at all. She told us to take gluten out of his diet, and then at the very next appointment she told us to put it back in. This is *not* how to go about dietary changes. Again, do your homework. Based on her initial recommendation, we got rid of all gluten the very next day. Have you ever witnessed a crack addict coming off of drugs? I haven't, but I am pretty sure it looks a lot like Rob did when he was coming off of wheat. He was acting like a lunatic. His pupils were dilated; he was erratic, irritable, and generally insane. I could not find a bread substitute that didn't taste like sand mixed with cardboard, so I baked my own loaf of gluten-free bread and made us sandwiches. Rob took one bite, got up, and grabbed the rest of the loaf. He put it on the floor, got on his hands and knees, and ate it like a dog. I had to find out what was going on with him.

I started reading Dr. Kenneth Bock's book *Healing the New Childhood Epidemics,* and a whole city's worth of light bulbs went on in my head. I learned about leaky gut and discovered that when gluten is digested, the peptides that remain from breaking down the protein mimic opiates. If your gut wall is damaged and permeable, these peptides can leave the gut, cross the blood brain barrier, and affect brain function. Rob was addicted to bread. Every piece he ate made him as high as a kite. I devoured Bock's book, started Rob on basic supplements, and at age five (on his and Jon's birthday), he went to a new DAN! doctor, who gave us a blueprint to start him on the road to recovery. I knew at once that this would take us no time at all, because when I decide to do something, I get it done. We were going to kick autism's ass up and down the block!

And so it began. We were running down the dream of recovery from autism. It is possible. I have actually watched it happen with a friend's son. Yet some of our kids—when you join the club you feel like every child and family affected is part of your family, too—are so sick and damaged that it feels like you are climbing a never-ending mountain, clawing your way to the top. We fell into that category. Around four years of age, Rob stopped growing and gaining weight. He just stopped. Not one of his doctors was concerned about this. Not our pediatrician, not our autism specialist, no one was as worried as we were about Rob's growth difficulties. I had to find answers on my own, so I booked an appointment with a pediatric gastroenterologist who specialized in autism.

Rob had profound failure to thrive. He "looked" healthy, but he was the size of a three- or four-year-old at age six. He weighed only thirty-one pounds. He was all bones when he took his shirt off but had a hard, distended belly most of the time. After our initial lab work and testing, the gastroenterologist found that there were markers for inflammation in the labs and said that we should consider a scope and a pill cam to investigate the inflammation. We traveled to his office and started the grueling process of getting our child scoped. Not feeding your already underweight child is a painful thing to do, but we knew we had to find out what was causing the lack of growth. The first step was the pill cam. Thankfully, Rob could swallow pills, so he just popped that capsule with the camera in his mouth, and down the hatch it went. He had to wear a backpack with monitoring equipment on him for the next six hours so it could record the pictures. Then we had to prep for the scope. Not only had this poor kid not eaten anything but we also had to make sure he was "cleaned out." We gave him laxatives and enemas, and boy did we clean him out! We headed to the surgical center the next day, got him ready to go, and then we waited. The procedure went well, and as expected, the doctor found inflammation in his small intestine that was similar to Crohn's disease. He also found abnormal cells in Rob's colon, which he said could have been a sign of previous inflammation.

Rob was happy and hungry after the procedure, and we could finally feed him. We started slowly introducing food and headed back to our hotel. That night, Rob started vomiting. We called our doctor, and he explained that sometimes that could happen when food is reintroduced. But it continued and didn't stop. A medication was called in to help stop the vomiting, but the next day the vomiting continued. Then he began throwing up bile. We went to the emergency room, and he was admitted. No one felt that the vomiting was caused by the scope, because he wasn't throwing up blood. However, they couldn't figure out what was happening either. An x-ray revealed that the pill cam did in fact pass, which is something they thought might have been causing the problem. The x-ray also showed that there was a mass in his abdomen that looked like a blood clot. He was having loads of tests done and was getting poked and prodded every ten minutes by someone from the hospital staff. The closest I have ever come to killing another human being was during the barium swallow. Rob would not drink this nasty stuff, so they had to put a tube down his nose to get the barium into his stomach. It was absolute torture for him, and I completely lost it on the staff. Jon was just sitting there, sobbing, while I was going mama bear on those poor technicians. Sweet Rob was lying there, crying and begging them to stop. It was hell. A hell I never want to see again. When we were finally discharged from the hospital a week later with almost no information about what had happened, Rob was skin and bones. The good news was that the mass in his abdomen was getting smaller, so it was just a blood clot and nothing we had to continue to worry about. Now we just had to get this GI problem solved and get this kid gaining weight. We started him on the medications that our doctor prescribed and hoped that this would be the answer we needed.

Every medication we put him on caused severe, debilitating migraines, and he still wasn't gaining weight. Our happy, sweet boy was in pain. Excruciating pain. He would grab his head and sob at breakfast, and he lost the sparkle in his eyes. We tried all of the medications over the course of nine months, and the same thing happened each time. The next step was a medication that would potentially alter his DNA, cause sterility, or possibly cancer. We decided then that we needed to find another solution. The solution was a new autism specialist, and this time we were not going to mess around. We were going to go to the best. We traveled to Florida. Once we got our road map from our new physician, we finally started to see some weight gain and much-needed growth. To this day, Rob remains extremely small for his age, and it weighs heavily on our minds.

We also found a classical homeopath who was experienced in autism. Since working with him, we have seen some nice changes in Rob, both physically and cognitively. We are continuing with these professionals currently and hope that, with their guidance and help, Rob will make great developmental strides. With each new intervention comes new hope that it will make a difference for our golden boy. We will continue the search and fight because recovery is possible.

I don't know if I will ever really know the full impact autism has had on our family, because I barely remember family life before autism. It has consumed our life for five years, and in some ways it has defined who each of us is. What autism takes from a family is incalculable. Autism takes everything. No matter what your station in life, if you are like us and believe that your child can recover from autism, it will cost you everything. You will spend all your time, money, and energy on it. It is worth every drop of blood, sweat, and tears because while autism has been transforming your child it has also been reshaping you. But your transformation is a change you have control over. You have choices about how you will adapt to this new life you are about to lead. You can become angry, negative and resentful. Actually, for a while you need to be. I needed a bit of denial. No, I needed a *lot* of denial. I needed to believe that Rob was fine, and there is a part of me that will always believe that. I have a big chunk of denial still in me. You need to cry, curled up in the fetal position with a bottle of wine and a box of chocolates. You need to throw things and scream. Then you need to decide what path you will take. What you do next is your choice. You can believe that this Goliath called autism is beatable, or you can decide that it is too big a challenge to face. For us the answer was always that we were going to come up swinging.

We have had our boxing gloves on for a long time now, and we are leaving no stone unturned. Something has happened to our child, and he is sick. We are going to find the answers that will make him well again. We have tried more interventions and therapies than I care to count. Speech, OT, ABA, RDI, HBOT, AIT, vision therapy, acupressure . . . the list is endless. All come with a hefty price tag attached. The medical list is even more extensive. Rob has endured more blood draws than anyone should ever have to deal with in a lifetime. He has had an MRI, an ambulatory EEG, a sleep-deprived EEG, and a bone age test. He has been scoped, which led to that horror of a hospitalization, and had a growth hormone challenge test. He has taken loads of daily supplements and had a fecal fat test (which I won't even go into) and countless appointments with specialists who can't, or won't, figure out how to help him. I wish there were more doctors out there who really and truly understand that our children are sick. Children are supposed to grow. They are supposed to develop on track, and when they don't, it means that something is wrong. It isn't "just autism," as so many of the physicians we go to looking for answers tell us. Our kids need help, and unfortunately the doctors who are willing and able to help them are few and far between and are in great demand.

Despite the uphill battle that we all have with the medical community in our efforts to help our children, there are people and programs that exist only to enrich the lives of kids with developmental disabilities. Thankfully, there are some amazing recreation programs out there for our kids. We have found a few great programs for Rob that we could not live without at this point. Rob is on a special-needs ice hockey team that he loves. It is an unbelievable program with exceptional families and wonderful mentors. Each week, high school hockey players from the area come to help Rob's team. They are kind and patient, and give up their Sunday afternoons to help kids with special needs learn to play hockey. Rob has blossomed since we joined this team, and we look forward to watching him grow as he learns more about hockey each day. It is a joy to watch all of the kids on his team have a blast for an hour and a half each week. For these moments I am grateful.

In fact, I feel blessed. I am fortunate. I am a lucky soul, and Rob certainly is too. It is not because I am someone who thinks that autism is a gift. It is not. Autism was handed to us in a pediatric exam room, and I would give anything to change that fact. We are blessed because we have the most amazing family and friends that anyone could ever ask for. The support that my family receives from our community is tremendous and, quite frankly, overwhelming to think about. I am on this road with the best kid on the planet, and he has a father and a brother who are up for the challenge of navigating this road with us. I am in awe daily of the person Rob's brother is becoming. At just six years old, he shows the world that he has more personality, heart, and compassion than most adults I know. I have watched him run off to play with a nonverbal child on the play-ground, and my heart swelled with pride. I have had my eyes well up watching him help Rob do something that is difficult for him. I have laughed at his silly jokes and larger-than-life personality. He is the most important friend, therapist, and playmate that Rob will ever have, and I am grateful every day that I got that second urge to have a baby. This ride would not be nearly as joyful without his infectious smile.

This brings me to Jon. I could write an entire book about my family, so where do I even begin with Jon? It feels as if we have been together for eternity. This is so cliché, but he really is my best friend. I am not sure that we would have made it this far if he weren't, because with autism every day brings new and exciting ways to strain a marriage to its breaking point. We are constantly worrying about paying for therapy, doctors' visits, and supplements in addition to all our "normal" monumental expenses. I am always researching, so Jon loses me to the computer for months at a time. Jon works horrific hours so he can keep advancing at work and keep the money coming in. I try to get as involved in the commu-nity as possible so that everyone knows and accepts Rob. This leads to my being overcommitted, which is something that drives Jon absolutely crazy. He doesn't like conflict. I am a fighter. Some days we are roommates at best. Other times we feel so ultraconnected and happy that it is like magic. The ups are wonderful, and the downs are like bottomless pits. But we love each other. We adore our kids. We love our life despite the "Big A" that has become a 500 lb. gorilla that follows us everywhere. We will make it work.

If you are reading this and just starting out, I will give you one piece of advice. Make time for your family . . . all of your family. Make time for your children without autism. They need you, too. Go out to lunch with them. Surprise them with a date for ice cream, even if you hate the idea of your kids even looking at sugar. Listen to their stories. Read with them. Praise them for their efforts with their sibling with autism. These warrior siblings are the most amazing people on the planet, and we need to nurture and encourage them so they can change the world. Above all, make time for your spouse. Your husband (or wife for all you male readers) is just as worried and stressed out as you are about your child. Be there for each other, and make time to remember why you even got married in the first place. Find something, one little thing, that you like to do together, and do it often. If you like to hike, make it a regular event. If you like to work in the yard, plant a garden. Find some common ground and make it work. It is a hell of a lot easier to offer this advice than it is to live it, and I am very guilty of not always honoring this rule.

While I am on the subject, I would like to take a moment to thank the Dave Matthews Band for saving our marriage. Maybe that is an exaggeration. I like to think our marriage didn't need saving, but we sure have had fun running around being wannabe groupies and acting like we are back in college again. We see the band a few times a year, and sometimes we get to travel to do it. For one blissful evening, we both forget all about autism and just have fun together. What could be better than a night away from home with no kids, a concert, a few beers, and the guy you love? Not much. So thanks, Dave!

For those of you reading who have children with autism, especially those of you who are just starting out, you cannot make it through this journey alone. You need support. Don't be afraid to ask for it! You may get some surprising help from a neighbor or an old friend. Take it. Don't turn down offers to help. Eventually, people will stop asking if you turn them down enough, and in my experience, people don't offer unless they mean it. You are going to be sad and angry at times. Get emotional support from your spouse if he or she is able and willing. I know that sometimes marriages just don't work out. Sadly, this is a common reality when faced with autism. It can wreak havoc on the happiest of homes, and it has done so in mine on occasion. If you can't count on your husband or wife for support, find some people you can lean on. You will have to put yourself out there in order to make this happen. Find a TACA meeting, get on a Yahoo! group, and find local families that are going through this, too. Get on Facebook if you haven't already. Seriously! The most amazing people are out there waiting with open arms to help you. They are your fellow autism parents. These fantastic moms and dads have been around the block a few times. They know their stuff and graciously hold out their hands and say, "We'll walk with you." I will forever be indebted to the amazing parents who have laughed with me, cried with me, and taught me so much about autism and life. They are the reason I have never given up. Find us. We are out there. Together we can do this.

I just know that someday sunshine will shoot out of all our kids' asses again.

Bytes from the Count

The biomed Dad. That's me. You know, I'm the one lone guy at a biomed meeting with ten ladies. I've met other biomed dads, but they only seem to know the basics. Once I start talking to them, they usually say their wives know more than they do. I think I have a one up on the biomed moms. Moms worry more about the child being in pain and are often reluctant to try some biomed things because of that. Dads are usually less fearful. Also, dads tend to call the shots more on financial matters.

All the dads are expected to keep their poker face on and tell the family everything's going to be all right. You panic, they'll lose all hope. I've had a day or two in which things were so down in the dumps with my son, I couldn't concentrate on anything at work. Had to walk and find a quiet stairwell to take a moment to cry. Then I got right back to my ultimate hack. If I ever hear another dad say he didn't have a moment like that, I don't believe him for a second.

★ ★ ★

I was in my bathroom. I looked in the mirror. And I stared at myself. "You piece of shit. You're a disgrace. What kind of life did you give your kids?" I felt sorry for myself. I looked pathetic. What did I ever do to anyone to deserve this? I don't know. But I'm going to make it right. And I hope I can look in the mirror one day and not be ashamed.

BLAZING A TRAIL TO RECOVERY

One sunny day when he was eight months old, I took my precious baby boy to the nursery at the YMCA. It was a great day to work out, and I was feeling motivated and positive.

After thirty minutes or so on the treadmill, I went to check on him. He was still in his car seat on the floor, and three or four little kids were hovering over him. They were trying to cheer him up because he was extremely upset and crying like a banshee on fire (please stop here and actually visualize a banshee on fire . . . I am not exaggerating). As I got closer, I saw that the kids' tactics were working a little. He would transition for a few seconds into maniacal laughter, but then, seamlessly and without a breath, he would go back to crying, as if in pain. Severe pain. A high-pitched belly laugh, then an inconsolable cry. Repeat.

This went on for a minute or so, and I sat down with the kids. At that moment, a woman walked by and said, "That child is bipolar, somebody needs to get that checked out," and kept on walking.

I was frozen. Bipolar is a scary word, and it was much more scary to me in that moment than it had ever been. I had recently witnessed bipolar behavior up close for the first time in my life when my husband's adopted brother lost his family and his home in a manic episode. I ran out of the YMCA as fast as I could and cried my eyes out all the way home, hyperventilating. I'm surprised I got us home safely. I was confused—and furious. I wanted to hunt down that woman and systematically ruin her life.

Years later, that day at the Y would be one of the few moments I could reach back to when I tried to remember what could have been a hint that something was going wrong with my son in his first year. I also remember my father playing with him and laughing that he just could not get Patrick to look him in the eye no matter what he did. Also in that first year, my boy had thrush and severe, constant diarrhea. He took four-hour naps and slept twelve hours a night. He was *superhuman* strong and acted violently when he didn't want to do something. I had to sit on him to brush his teeth, to cut his nails, and to get him into his car seat. Getting him out of the pool, off the beach, and into a store was like World War III. My whole family thought he was a genius because he could label colors, shapes, letters, and numbers at eighteen months, but he had never put two words together. He was a first child and grandchild, and for some reason, no one around me really thought much of these things. Neither did I. And as it went, ignorance was bliss for almost three years.

Sam and I had been married for five years. I was thirty-three when I got pregnant. We were ready for kids. As far as pregnancies go, it wasn't all that interesting, exciting as it was for our families. I was extremely nauseous (so much so that I had to leave my job) and craved sugar like it was crack, but otherwise, it was a relatively uneventful pregnancy. Labor started two weeks after Patrick's due date, and I had thirty-five miserable hours of it. Friends and family were in the room after he was born, and I screamed at the mothers in the crowd that they were liars! Childbirth was far more painful than I expected; I had four doses of epidural meds, and that still didn't even touch the pain. (Afterwards, I realized that the excruciating pain I had in my pelvic area was from the fact that Patrick was breaking my tailbone as he moved through. Like many women are told to do by their doctors, I was lying flat on my back during delivery. I understand now that if you sit up, your tailbone moves out of the way. I also understand that it is an insurance issue. Thanks.)

I didn't sit for six months after Patrick was born and can still feel the injury eleven years since then. Later, I was worried about what it might have done to his head, but an MRI at age four showed nothing concerning.

The day came when the pediatrician told me that I should take Patrick to a speech therapist. I was floored. Really? A neighborhood acquaintance had been a speech therapist before she had children, so I asked her for advice. Though I know now that she probably didn't tell me what she really thought, she said that the general rule is a child should put two words together by age two, and three words together by age three. This was three months before Patrick's third birthday, and he had not put two words together. Ever.

The appointment was made, and twenty minutes into it the therapist said Patrick had pervasive developmental disorder (PDD). I immediately scooped up my son and walked out without a question. How dare you label my child, you scum! I didn't know what she meant by pervasive developmental disorder, nor did I care. I was five months pregnant and about to round out my perfect little family with a baby girl. Everything was fine, even if I was told by my OB to stay home for fear that my firstborn's extreme tantrums would make me miscarry.

I stewed on the therapist's diagnosis for six hours. When I couldn't sleep that night, I got up and googled PDD. I learned what it really meant. Autism. There it was in black and white. I had heard of autism, but I was mistaken in thinking I had not seen it with my own eyes. I was terrified. Autism. Would my new baby have it, too?

I hit the ground running immediately after the diagnosis. The first thing I found out was that if a kid eats only wheat and dairy, there are probably going to be good results when you take those foods away. We got great results, but what we went through to get them was no picnic. Imagine following your diapered toddler around the house for twelve straight nighttime hours while he wanders from corner to corner dry-heaving from withdrawal. It took everything I had not to shove a Cheerio down his throat. But after three days without the cheese quesadillas, yogurt, goldfish, bread, cereal, and pasta that I had allowed him to narrow himself down to, he looked at me. I mean, really looked at me. Up and down, with wonder, as if he'd never seen me before. As if the blindfold had been taken off and he could actually see the person who was caring for him. That was all I needed to see.

The thing that happens to some of us, though, is that if you find an intervention that helps your child, you want to know why it's working. Why did the diet help my child? Was it because heavy metals from his substantial amount of childhood vaccines killed his digestive enzymes in his stomach, so proteins in certain foods did not get digested properly? This set off a whole new world of research and shock for me.

Here is what I found: He had the hepatitis B (Hep B) vaccine in the hospital at birth and one each at six months, nine months, and fifteen months (this is one more than is recommended by the CDC). Each of these shots had 25 mcg of thimerosal (a preservative half of which is mercury; a neurotoxin). They were the only shots he had that contained more than a trace amount of thimerosal. That dosage, 25 mcg, is more than is allowed by the EPA for a 550 lb. adult. My research has also led me to believe that aluminum exposure from his vaccines also affected Patrick along with the sheer stress to his immune system of receiving four vaccines in one day every two months. Today, there are often more than four vaccines given to kids in one day.

I found that if you treat the body for vaccine injury-related conditions (including inflammation, enzyme deficiencies, rogue viruses, bacteria, and fungi), then symptoms of autism could improve. But wait a minute! The media, the doctors, our community—they all say this is impossible. Disproven. Ridiculous. Crazy.

What I'm here to say is that we are *not* crazy. Vaccines may not be a trigger for every child's autistic symptoms, but they certainly were for my child. The proof is in his improvement as we've treated him for vaccine injury.

As far as I am concerned, there are a few aspects about the vaccine/autism story that are ignored: First of all, the vaccines that children receive today are not studied for their effects in combination with one another. Some components have not been tested for safety at all. Many in the medical field do not seem to understand that if a child has a compromised immune system (either from genetics or from an illness), vaccines may not work as planned. As a patient advocate at my pediatrician's office, I did intake on about 300 families, most of whom reported a family history of immune dysfunction. My son's grandmothers both have lupus, and my sister spent a week in the hospital after receiving the MMR when she was seven. How can you "trick" an immune system with a vaccine (which contains the disease it's supposed to protect from) when that immune system is already challenged? Any number of problems can result from that scenario.

I initially found the information I needed to help Patrick on the Internet. A few books like Karen Serrousi's *Unraveling the Mystery of Autism and Pervasive Developmental Disorder* and Jacqueline McCandless's *Children with Starving Brains* told stories that fit my family like a glove. I treated Patrick with diet and supplements carefully picked by my own extensive research. Doctors who knew about this approach were hard to come by, and the good ones had waiting lists over a year. The big miracle came when we were able to get an appointment with a world-renowned autism specialist in Florida, a few hours away from us in Georgia. The ball started rolling when we convinced a local integrative pediatrician to help administer IVs to pull out the heavy metals, get us into a hyperbaric chamber, and fine-tune his treatment plan.

Obviously, autism advocacy isn't what I planned for my life. I was president of the Student Council and of the illegal "sorority" in high school. I went on scholarship to a private college and transferred to the best state school and did the sorority-girl thing. After graduating, I anchored my hometown news for a while before I moved to the big city to work in TV and telecommunications.

Looking back, I suppose all of it put together gave me the skills and determinations to be what I needed to be for my son. As an autism parent, you become a researcher whether you like it or not. Leadership skills are a plus for managing caseworkers, doctors, therapists, the state, and insurance companies. In my case, I also became an investigator. Finding the real story of autism and sharing it with the media and the world became my life. Not all autism moms become activists or advocates, but that's where this journey has taken me.

It is nothing short of mind-blowing to watch the activists in the autism world and read their writings. Their stories and commitment inspired me, and I wanted to be among them. When our son was four and our daughter was one, we marched on Washington, D.C. in protest of the current recommended childhood vaccine schedule. I got involved with our local autism nonprofit and served on the board. We held walks, went to conferences, gave money to families, helped other parents in the school setting with IEPs. I sat in on meetings to get the school system up to speed on how to serve our children. I signed up as a rescue angel to help other families through Generation Rescue. I contacted media and went on the news to talk about Dr. Wakefield's MMR paper, the Supreme Court's role in whether pharma can be sued for vaccine injury, my son's progress, and a mercury spill at his school. I was quoted in the newspaper about vaccine requirements for school. I was named "Woman to Watch" by a local magazine and "Champion of Change" by a local TV station.

I talked my pediatrician into hiring me to counsel families on how to help their children change their diet, do testing to find answers, and get help in the community. I also convinced him to admit on local TV that vaccines caused my son's autism. The next morning, the clip circled back around to me from Australia! I helped organize a local art show to raise money for Generation Rescue. I have spoken at the CDC and was asked to head my state in the newly formed Canary Party, a group of citizens concerned about the health of our nation.

But all that activism has taken its toll on my personal life. Sometimes I get so wrapped up in wanting things to change, for the people in charge to realize things have gone way wrong with our healthcare and our corporate greed, that things fall apart. I've drunk way too much alcohol and have at times completely lost my path with my husband. I was diagnosed with fibromyalgia and took way too many prescription pills for pain. I gained thirty pounds. My parents had no idea what to do with me, so they distanced themselves. They did not want to encourage my fear and negativity, so instead of comforting me and endorsing my behavior, they decided to stay away. I lost friends, not just over differences in opinion about vaccines but over what they called my narrow and negative view of life. I preferred to think of myself as frightened, but there was truth in their observations of me: Autism was it. All there was for me. All I could talk about.

I spent many nights in the garage, talking for hours with mothers like me, devising plans, discussing the pros and cons of foods and doctors and supplements and medications and treatments on a list a hundred miles long. This is all on top of actually caring for my son, making sure his school environment was safe, making sure he got to the doctors and therapists, that he didn't eat the wrong foods, that he got twenty supplements a day, and that his bottom was clean until he was six years old. His behaviors and tantrums and resistance caused me to injure my back several times, and once there was a kick to the head bad enough to require a CT scan.

So things have been stressful. Times have been tough. But I struggle and mostly succeed in keeping it positive. I credit my husband with keeping us laughing and the mood light. Even though Sam and I have had our different ways of grieving, he is the best father and mate I could have possibly asked for in this situation. Our ups and our downs will always end on an "up." He is so patient, spending countless hours working on art projects and homework with our son. He keeps us stocked up on waffles made from grains he mills himself. He organized a fundraiser that raised half of the money for our county's Project Lifesaver system, a tracking system for children and adults who wander. When he raised that money, our child didn't even need it anymore! He did it for the community. He loves me no matter how fat or crazy or overzealous I am and has allowed me full control over our son's medical treatment with 100 percent support.

Not many autism families work as a team as well as we do, and I am so grateful. I do my best to not take my husband for granted, even when I'm feeling overwhelmed with cooking gluten-free meals *plus* the gluten-filled ones that the rest of us want. He works for my dad in our family business, and though my parents and I have our differences in opinion on how much I need to be involved in this cause, they have made every effort financially to support Patrick's therapies and diet (have you seen the prices of organic eggs?!).

Speaking of money, I cannot even count how much we have spent. One hundred hours of hyperbaric treatments, a sauna for the garage, a thousand-dollar water filter, special food for every single meal, trips to Florida to visit the doctor, plus a huge chunk for a behavioral therapy that required a new computer, a video camera and an out-of-state therapist. And I never even followed through on that one (insert sound of a toilet flushing here . . .).

Social skills groups . . . a top-notch homeopath . . . therapy for my husband and I . . . it's endless. We ran through the savings and 401(k)s from our previous lives in the corporate world in year one, then piled up a $23,000 mountain of credit card debt before the end of the next.

So all this work, all this stress, all this illness and tragedy and cost . . . where has it gotten us? Well, I have good news. Our son has gone from a violent, disconnected toddler to a fully included fifth grader without academic accommodation. He has had four pieces of his artwork hanging in local museums. He entertains himself and us by copying the online cartoon tutorials to a T in one sitting. We enjoy ourselves as a family.

Lots of people ask about what Patrick eats, since his diet is wheat- and dairy-free and we try to keep away from soy. He likes eggs, rice cakes, nut butters, bananas, apples, meats, French fries, and "safe" pizza (our local pizza joint serves pretty good gluten-free alternative, yay!). I can definitely get vegetables into Patrick with a little salt. We keep pesticide and other toxins to a minimum by buying organic food whenever possible and using natural cleaning products. When life begins to creep in and his diet rules get lax, we notice less and less of the unpleasant behaviors. We have been using homeopathy since last year, and this has contributed to finding more balance.

Today, we live with a high-functioning child who lies on the cusp of an Asperger's syndrome diagnosis. He tells stories all day that are usually straight from a movie plot. He and his neurotypical sister have a great relationship, and we revel in their frequent sibling bickering and rivalry (that's typical, right!?). He still takes the stairs one by one coming down and has reading comprehension issues (that we have found to be convergence issues with his eyes). He is sensitive to sunlight. He battles with yeast and strep that affect his bowels and behavior. He cannot participate in team sports.

He is sweet as pie, and when he gets in trouble, he is truly worried about it. He's constantly creating things (even if it is out of trash, which drives me crazy!). He is great at math and well liked in his class. He loves to swim. He has a beautiful singing voice, and his teachers think the next thing he should get involved with is children's theater.

Patrick wouldn't be where he is today without the intelligent, compassionate, brilliant people who have shown up in our lives. I credit his current pediatrician and staff, our specialist in Florida, numerous teachers and therapists, a huge crowd of *amazing* autism mothers (see all previous chapters of this book to start), and my family for his incredible strides. In the bigger picture, there are parents and doctors who came before me and set the trail on fire so that I could find the information I needed.

It's impossible to know what the future holds for my son. Middle school, puberty, increasingly complicated social situations, and just plain old mother's worry hang over my head daily. Though we have come far, we are not done with autism. But we are close to it becoming another part of our lives rather than the center of it. Regardless of where we end up, I am totally willing to accept him for who he is. All I want is for him to be happy and a productive member of society.

We will keep working and striving for him to have everything he needs to make it in this life. So many of us are helping the world become more and more cognizant of the different personality types that are flooding our society. While I make sure my son keeps growing, I will keep on marching and reaching out and speaking up.

While I love my son and I'm stronger for being an autism mom, I'm still not happy about it. I do not believe that God gave Patrick to me because he thought I was special and could handle a special child. Any God I would believe in wouldn't hurt a child to teach me a lesson. Don't send me that email. The one about how I have landed in Holland instead of Italy either. My friends from Holland don't appreciate that one at all!

The truth as I see it is that greed has poisoned our children, plain and simple. My son is a victim of greed, the motivating force behind a pharmaceutical industry that profits from making people sick so it can sell more meds that make us sicker. But people are writing about their experiences and talking and taking control of their families' health, and things are going to change. And this person that I have become won't shut up until they do.

EPILOGUE

So, where are the Thinking Moms now?

The majority of our book was written in late 2011 through the summer of 2012. As you can imagine, things have changed: our kids have gotten older, our group has gotten closer, and we have started a revolution online. Our daily blog (www.thinkingmomsrevolution. com) turned into more than just a blog. It's a platform, our voice, an outlet, a resource, and a chance to connect with you. The blog and our Facebook page (www.facebook.com/thinkingmomsrevolution) is the best way to keep up with us—what we are doing, who we are talking to, and where we hope to be.

At the same time, some things stayed the same. Several of our kids are still very sick; some of us are still fighting the same school battles. Some days are really good, and some days remain very difficult. Because of that and because a number of our children are getting better, healthier, and yes, closer to recovery, we will continue this great effort, this necessary movement, and one of the most important missions of our lives—a revolution like no other. As always, because we want more than just the best for all of our children, we ask you to join us, walk with us hand in hand, and go forward together into a future full of hope.

ACKNOWLEDGMENTS

We, the members of The Thinking Moms' Revolution (TMR), would like to express our sincere gratitude to the following individuals for their priceless assistance and support of our efforts in writing this book. Their unwavering tenacity and tireless efforts to help us create change and heal our children inspire us daily.

We are honored to walk among you and wouldn't be where we are today without you. We are truly grateful for your belief that we can be a part of the revolution to reclaim the health of our world's children.

We would like to acknowledge Dan Olmsted, Cathy Brazeal, Brooke Dougherty, Jenny McCarthy, Ed and Teri Arranga, Laura Rowley, Jacey Capurso, Louise Habakus, Kim Stagliano, Curt and Kim Linderman, Heidi Stevenson, Marcella Piper-Terry, the founders of AIM (Autism Is Medical) Jeanna Reed, Mandee Lochbaum, and Jill Rubolino, Michael Belkin, Lujene Clark, Anne Dachel, Jessica Gianelloni, Dr. Jeff Bradstreet, Candace McDonald, Monique Peltz, Stephanie Rotondi, Zeynel Karcioglu, Pierre Fontaine, Recovering Nicholas, and Tony Lyons and the team at Skyhorse for exactly those reasons.

A nod to the Turds as well (you know who you are), especially Jerry, our Ripple in Still Water.

Of course, our families deserve the most credit. They have allowed us to spend our extra (and not so extra) time on this project and have supported us all the way. Husbands, wife, siblings, and parents were there supporting us while we spent endless hours on Facebook and Skype working to make this happen, and for that we could not be more grateful. Our love knows no bounds.

And last but not least, TMR wouldn't exist if it weren't for Mark Zuckerberg. We would not have met and come together in this fashion. To quote our favorite *Texan*, "Facebook *is* important!" ;)

About Us

B.K., Booty Kicker (Melanie Baldwin)—I'm a mom to a ten-year-old son with autism who has self-injurious behaviors. I was diagnosed with breast cancer in February 2010, so now I'm kicking breast cancer *and* autism's booty! I have a lot on my plate, but my faith as a Christian is what gets me through. That and the support from some amazing friends.

Blaze (Kim Spencer)—I'm just a Southern girl trying to raise 2 beautiful kids . . . one with PANDAS and high-functioning autism. I believe with all my heart that if we can save *one* child from the fate of human-induced health problems, we can save the *world*! Things I love include the hubby, the Avett Brothers, old convertible Bugs, and Revolution!

Cupcake (Angele O'Connell)—I'm the girl from ChiTown with all the guy friends growing up . . . and am still surrounded by boys—my husband and two sons. My oldest is the king of everything and suffered from misdiagnosis after misdiagnosis until he was vaccine injured and our lives spiraled down into the world of autism. His little brother is my champion and keeps me going every day. He's in perfect health even though he has a hypogam diagnosis. My friends think I'm as sweet as a cupcake, but doctors and our former school district call me by a different name. Because of that school district, I—Bears fan—now live in enemy territory so my boys can get a proper and *safe* education. I am only as strong as my foundation, and that foundation is made up of my husband and two boys. They give me strength to heal my family and to prove to the doctors that yes, he *can* get better.

Dragon Slayer (Marissa Bagshaw)—I am a mother of two daughters who are recovered from autism. I read Sci-Fi/Fantasy and paranormal chick-lit (don't judge!). I love to travel and am a self-confessed shoes and handbag-aholic—I bask in the glory that is Chanel. In real-life, I'm covered in crumbs, boogers, and barf. My favorite topics of conversation includes methylation, candida, and poop. I'm working on it. I live in Malaysia with my husband and two daughters. I slay metaphorical dragons on a daily basis.

Goddess (Helen Conroy)—Mama of three cuties that I *adore* and really into Healing Harry, my sweet four-year-old who has autism. I am obsessed with autism research and staying on top of everything new treatment-wise (but not necessarily being the first to try it) while trying to juggle working full time and three different school schedules. I am passionate about supporting newly diagnosed families, and if you fit that category and are reading this, *there is hope—don't let anyone tell you otherwise*! I am extremely grateful for my hubby, our awesome extended family, and all their help. I am happily distracted by sunglasses, wine, and Facebook . . . and by little blue Tiffany boxes.

Luv Bug (Cathleen Reilly)—Born and bred city girl currently living in Who-ville. My ten-year-old son has autism and dwarfism and can escort you through any city subway system—no prob. My seven-year-old daughter is an amazing collector of Barbies and stuffed animals. She deals with her own chronic health issues as an afterthought. Me, not so much. DH and I run our businesses from a converted clam shack behind our home, while our two long-haired cats hide toddler-sized tufts of hair in every available corner. Life isn't tidy, but it's always interesting—and filled with love.

Mama Bear (Judi Tandari)—The name says it all. I am fiercely protective of my three children, especially my son Nicholas. I can be your best friend or your worst enemy. I can give you a bear hug or a bear claw . . . your choice. I have chosen to be a friend to the amazing parents who share this journey of healing with me, and an enemy to autism and those who try to prevent us from reaching our goal. When I'm not in battle (or at a sporting event for my kids), I enjoy shoes, scarves, and underwear (yeah, yeah . . . not in an exciting sort of way). I believe that when determined parents unite, nothing is impossible. There is no greater motivation than the love we feel for our children. We will be victorious!!!!!!

Mama Mac (Alison Macneil)—Alison MacNeil, you've met my family on the *Autism Now* series on PBS last spring. Continue with me as I work hard at healing Nick's mind and body, gently guiding my typically developing daughter through the trials of middle school, and pushing for change in the politics of autism every day.

Mamacita (Cathy Jameson)—Flowing through life with a hint of spice. I'm crunchy, salty, zingy, nibbly, and yet comforting. Always willing to give the benefit of the doubt before pouncing, I have stepped on a few toes righting wrongs that have harmed my child. My son is nonverbal, yet aching to talk. Until he does, I don't mind speaking up for him.

Money (Monika Ostroff)—Mom to a beautiful five-year-old girl with an infectious laugh and impish sense of humor who also happens to have ASD. Optimism, humor, hope, love, and laughter carry us all along the path to her full recovery. I'm thankful every day for meeting this amazing group of parents who have become such an incredible source of strength, support, and knowledge. But enough about me; let's get on with healing our kids!!

Mountain Mama (Cam Baker Pearson)—I was born in the summer of my thirty-second year when I came "home" to Montana. I am the proud mother of two beautiful little boys (one ASD, one NT) and the wife of an amazing man and father. In the spring and summer, you will find me shovel in hand, knee deep in soil in our organic garden. In the winter, you will find me shovel in hand, knee deep in the snow. No matter the season, I wield a metaphorical shovel, beating back toxic insults, seizures, Tourette's, bad medical practices, and anyone who stands in the way of my son reaching his full potential. In a former life, I enjoyed literary analysis, teaching English, and photojournalism. Now, I enjoy nature walks, the laughter of my boys, and torturing my family with the musical stylings of John Denver.

Poppy—Mother of two boys with ASD working toward recovery every single day. NYC born and raised, I now live at the beach. I'm rough around the edges and says what's on my mind. I'm sick of bad food, bad medicine, bad vaccines, bad water, bad business, and bad politics, and I'm ready to rattle some cages and make some changes. . . .

Prima (Claire V. Chriqui)—"Frenchie" by last name, I was born and raised across the sea. I believe that a life without cause is a life without effect. I am the proud mom of two miracle children. My dream and my cause are to heal my beautiful son, who is medically fragile, with a resume of autoimmune and neurological conditions. But despite the seriousness of this statement, I still try to have fun doing it . . . What's life without good (healthy) food, good (healthy?!?) wine, good music, a little fashion here and there—and a dream to one day wear again those dancing shoes!!! Dreams are not negotiable in this house. You can only live once, but if you do it right, once is enough!

Princess (Leia Michal)—I'm mom to two beautiful boys, one of whom (my five-year-old) a nonverbal angel with autism. In addition to pursuing biomedical interventions to address my son's medical challenges, I've discovered that although I can't control autism, I can control how I respond to it. I have found a deep comfort and happiness by choosing to see everything in our life as an opportunity and as a result, and I have been privileged to be a part of an extremely spiritual journey with my son. My life now feels filled with blessing as I get to partake in the deepening and blossoming of my relationship with my son. I believe that, ultimately, love will be a huge piece of his recovery. In my spare time, I enjoy design and beading, and if you're ever looking for someone to eat with, I'm the ultimate foodie!

Professor (Zoey O'Toole)—Quirky actor/geek with a degree in physics and a lifelong interest in autism. I am a mystery reader who, like The Count, has a deep-seated need to solve puzzles. I have a twelve-year-old Renaissance woman in the making with ADHD and a five-year-old future architect who *used* to have apraxia. I owe the fact that my kids do *not* have autism to other parents who have been generous with their experience and information. This is my chance to pay it forward.

Saint (Jennifer Limekiller)—You know the story about the person walking down the beach and saving starfish? Well, that is me, except my goal is to save children. I am a school psychologist by day who strives to save high school students from their past, their environment, and oftentimes, themselves. I then come home to my other full-time job, the one that pays me with unconditional love and unlimited hugs. I am a single mom to my beautiful fourteen-year-old adopted daughter who actually picked me out ten years ago when I was attempting to save her biological family. More on that in my chapter, but the four years of neglect she suffered before we met, along with prenatal abuse, left my girl with numerous disabilities and medical conditions. She is my greatest blessing and does not deserve what life has handed her. I will not stop until I make that right.

Savage (Bridgette Selvaggio)—Polish/Italian wife, mother to two wonderful kids, and as the name implies, "a force of nature." I am passionate about organic and sustainable farming practices, non-GMO food, and holistic living. After my son's diagnosis of autism at age three, it became imperative to me to become educated about the harmful effects of toxins in our food, water, and environment and how this has led to skyrocketing diagnoses of autoimmune dysfunction, asthma, learning disorders, and autism. When I'm not making green smoothies, I'm usually watching the *Real Housewives*.

Snap (Jill Bellestri)—I'm a Sagittarius, and I like long walks in the park and cooking. Not really . . . I would rather be driven around in a limo and have a personal chef. I have a wonderful husband as long as he is doing what I tell him to do, and we have a beautiful ten-year-old son affected by autism. My son is smart, funny, and adorable. My mission in life is that no matter how long or how much effort it takes, I will beat autism. I wake up every day fighting autism, and I will not stop. One of my favorite quotes is by Martin Luther King: "Our lives begin to end the day we become silent about the things that matter." A message to the naysayers: autism matters to me, and I will never be silent.

Sugah—A dry-witted southerner working fiercely to kick some autism a$$. Sassy. Independent. Strong minded. I am passionate about Jesus and healing my family. I will *nevah give up*!

Sunshine (Megan Davenhall)—Lone girl in a house of boys. Life is practically perfect in every way! Oh, except for this pesky autism that just showed up one day. My husband and I work tirelessly to help our beautiful boy shed his diagnosis and shine like the star he was born to be (when we aren't running around after DMB that is). You just watch what happens! Together the two of us can move mountains.

Tex (Thalia Seggelink)—*Yippeee kai yay* and *yeeeeeeee haaaaawww*!!!!! This pistol-packin' mama hails from Austin, Texas, . . . and Seattle . . . and Atlanta . . . and Baton Rouge . . . and Panama City, Panama. Though I clearly got my nickname based on my current residence, I'd like to think it has more do with my "Wild West" attitude. I'm a crunchy conservative in love with God, family, and my juicer. (Yummmm!!!!) My boy/girl twins are my inspiration and passion. I spend my days trying to tame the bucking bronco of my son's autism and enjoying the gallop that has become my life.

My message is simple: if you want to do something badly enough, you'll *find* a way. Whatever you do, don't drink the Haterade!!!!

The Count (Sunil Patel)—Who, me? . . . The lone dude here? . . . I'm just an engineer. I solve puzzles for a living. The same day my son got his diagnosis, I searched for more information. It was also the same day I realized this problem was solvable. Every one of our kids has a unique problem, and for each there's a unique answer. Come with me on my quest! Watch me go full circle as I move toward the end. But first, if you don't mind, let's stop at a bar. We're going to need some fuel for the journey.

The Rev (Lisa Joyce Goes)—I am a mom to three amazing children, one of whom suffers greatly with mitochondrial dysfunction, bowel disease, and immune compromise—all serious medical conditions that were mistakenly diagnosed as autism. I am managing partner at The Misuta Project, an autism media company in search of the truth and in support of those pursuing it. I'm also a contributing editor for *Age of Autism* and executive board member of the Illinois Canary Party. I frequently guest blog for the U.S. Autism and Asperger's Association, New Day Autism Foundation, and Adventures in Autism. Clearly, I am the Rev because I cannot stop preaching the *truth*! Which (big sigh of relief) you will find *here*. Welcome!

Twonk (Jai Power)—About me? Ummm . . . I'm mostly sane, slightly damaged, from West London . . . trying not to stand out like a tourist in the American South.

OUR FAVORITE RESOURCES

Adventures in Autism: http://adventuresinautism.blogspot.com/
Age of Autism: www.ageofautism.com/
Anne Dachel: www.annedachel.com/
AutismOne: www.autismone.org/
Autism Aid: www.autismaid.org/
Autism Is Medical: www.meetup.com/Autism-Is-Medical/
Autism Research Institute:www.autism.com/
Elizabeth Birt Center for Autism Law & Advocacy: www.ebcala.org/
Gaia Health: www.gaia-health.com/
Generation Rescue: www.generationrescue.org/
Linderman Unleashed: http://radio.naturalnews.com/
    Archive-LindermanUnleashed.asp
National Autism Association: http://nationalautismassociation.org/
National Vaccine Information Center: www.nvic.org/
Natural News Radio: http://radio.naturalnews.com/
Regarding Caroline: http://regardingcaroline.com/
Safeminds: www.safeminds.org/
Surfers for Autism: www.surfersforautism.org/
Surfers Healing: www.surfershealing.org/
Talk About Curing Autism: www.tacanow.org/
The Autism File: www.autismfile.com/
The Bolen Report: www.bolenreport.com/
The Canary Party: :www.canaryparty.org/

The Misuta Project: www.youtube.com/user/ljactivist
The Puzzling Piece: www.thepuzzlingpiece.com/
The Refusers: http://therefusers.com/
The Sears Family: http://askdrsears.com
Vactruth: http://vactruth.com/
Vaxtruth: http://vaxtruth.org/

INDEX